Flesh & Blood

ALSO BY N. WEST MOSS

The Subway Stops at Bryant Park: Stories

Flesh & Blood

Reflections on Infertility, Family, and Creating a Bountiful Life

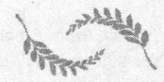

N. West Moss

ALGONQUIN BOOKS OF
CHAPEL HILL 2021

Published by
Algonquin Books of Chapel Hill
Post Office Box 2225
Chapel Hill, North Carolina 27515-2225

a division of
Workman Publishing
225 Varick Street
New York, New York 10014

The short story "Because His Wife" is from Grasses and Trees
by A. L. Snijders, translated by Lydia Davis. Published by
AFdH Publishers, the Netherlands, 2016.

Thanks to McSweeney's Internet Tendency, which first published "Things to
Discuss with My Doctor Before the Hysterectomy" in 2016.

Library of Congress Cataloging-in-Publication Data

Names: Moss, N. West (Nanette West), [date]– author.
Title: Flesh & blood / N. West Moss.
Other titles: Flesh and blood
Description: Chapel Hill, North Carolina : Algonquin Books of
Chapel Hill, 2021. | Summary: "A deeply personal memoir
on illness and infertility"— Provided by publisher.
Identifiers: LCCN 2021019228 | ISBN 9781643750705 (hardcover) |
ISBN 9781643752204 (ebook)
Subjects: LCSH: Moss, N. West (Nanette West), [date]—Health. |
Infertility, Female—Patients—United States—Biography. | Miscarriage—
Psychological aspects. | Pregnancy—Psychological aspects.
Classification: LCC RG201 .M68 2021 |
DDC 618.1/780092 [B]—dc23
LC record available at https://lccn.loc.gov/2021019228

10 9 8 7 6 5 4 3 2 1
First Edition

For my mother
and her mother
and her mother
and *her* mother

Contents

Part Three: At the Hospital for Surgery

Flesh & Blood

Prologue

I was six years old when Grandma Hastings died, at the end of the year she came to live with us. The night before her funeral, my mother rolled my hair around plastic curlers, which pressed painfully into my scalp as I tried to sleep. My father said that at Grandma's funeral I cried like an adult, real sobs of comprehending grief. My mother remembers that I went from ashtray to ashtray at the church gathering spent matches, then sat cross-legged under a table eating the burnt match heads, acting out some inexplicable ritual of mourning, the sulfur crumbling on my tongue. Ashes to ashes.

Even before I got married and put her wedding ring permanently on my finger, Grandma Hastings was with me. For a lifetime now I've thought of her as I fell asleep at night. When my mother reads to me, I hear my grandmother's soft voice. Grandma Hastings is with me when I write, when I mourn the loss of my own unborn children, when I walk in the woods, when I visit New Orleans. She is with me, hardly perceptible but there like the air, like the unnoticed but vital pull of gravity.

We do not always choose who walks with us, who we will find ourselves leaning on in times of duress. I only understand this in retrospect, long after the story I'm about to tell, long after the illness, diagnosis, and recovery are behind me. I woke up one morning and thought: *Grandma Hastings has been beside me all this while. How much harder this would have been without her.*

I have a writing room, an office called Beside the Point. It's up in the attic where the world can't interrupt me. There is a chair there that I bought at a thrift store for $9.99. It is large and comfortable and piled with books and papers, but now and then I clear it off as an invitation for Grandma Hastings, a woman who briefly, when I was almost six years old, opened up worlds for me. I like to imagine her sitting with me while I work.

Part One

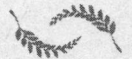

Pre-Diagnosis

ONE

Blood

exsanguinate (ek-sang′gwi-nāt): 1. To remove or with-
draw the circulating blood; to make bloodless

—TheFreeDictionary.com

At fifty-two I am old to still be bleeding so much,
but my body is a stranger to me. The blood
flows, insistent as a river, dragging me from my bed at
night, over and over. Messes to clean up in the dark. My
strength pouring out of me. For months and months and
months, I have been bleeding a lot. How can I *have* this
much blood? How can there be more?

When will it end?

Will it *ever* end?

ALREADY AN AUTHOR, I've decided to take an advanced
writing class at the school in New Jersey where I am an
adjunct professor, and I wear a pretty dress because I am

happy to be in this class with a teacher I love, happy to be writing.

The dress is from Old Navy and is white with tiny flowers scattered over it. Because of all the blood, I am also wearing a super plus tampon, and a maxi pad, the biggest they make. My body and I are two different entities now, and I don't know what to expect, like it's an unreliable child I'm bringing along who might need snacks or to be reprimanded, might be charming or throw a tantrum. All I am sure of is this body is unpredictable.

So, beneath my dress I have my gauzy armor in place when the professor says, after several hours of class, "Let's take a ten-minute break," and classmates begin to rustle around me, stretching and gathering up their papers.

Time slows as I stand up and blood just spills out of me, right through the super plus tampon, right over the sides of the enormous pad. It travels down the length of my thighs, over the hills of my knees, past my shins and the knobs of my ankles, and within less than a second, it starts to puddle beneath the arches of my feet inside my shoes.

I'm sure that everyone has seen and is horrified. (I find out later that no one noticed anything—a lesson

I've had to learn over and over again, that no one is ever looking at me, as much as I dread and hope that they are.) I take my bag and walk quickly, without making a noise, to the nearest bathroom (which happens to belong to the dean of the college). I go as fast as a person can with her legs pressed together. I'm shaking. My feet are squishing in the blood that's filling my shoes.

On the toilet I feel clots coming out of me and it reminds me of that big second-trimester miscarriage from years ago. But now there's no cramping, no panting. The blood clots are so large, though, that I can feel them like islands in a river. There is an enormous amount of blood—an alarming amount. There is blood all over my legs. Blood on the floor.

I spit on wads of toilet paper and scrub my ankles and thighs. I bunch up the toilet paper and then paper towels between my legs and wash my shoes in the sink, and then I get on my hands and knees and clean the floor, trembling, quiet as a mouse.

Because this is the dean's bathroom, and because this is all happening at a school where I slid from visiting professor to lecturer to adjunct, and where I'd like a real, permanent job one day (that I won't ever get), the complexity of the situation dumbfounds me, telescopes away from me into outer space.

It occurs to me as I frantically clean that I have spent a lot of my life cleaning up after myself in fear and shame. I think too about how my uterus and I have been at odds for forever. It has given me a lot of work and mess and worry over the decades, and for what? No children to show for the years of late-night trips back and forth to the bathroom, for the in-the-dark sinks full of cold water, for all the ruined mattresses, thrown away underwear, interrupted sleep.

A tear falls into the blood on the floor and makes a little clear spot through which I can see the white tile. I feel too old for this. I feel too old for everything. It would be nice to lie down on the cool tile floor, I think, press my cheek against its chilly face, to just give up and rest. Soldiering on feels beyond my capacity. Horizontal seems much more peaceful than vertical, and I feel the floor pulling me down. But no. As my shaking hands wipe up blood from the tile, my mind begins to plan what to do next.

Plan, plan, plan.

I left my phone at home (god, I'm disorganized), so I can't call my husband, and I won't go back into class now and ask for help. It's too embarrassing and frightening with my legs all bloody, and if I go in now and make a scene, I'll never be able to look at any of them again, and this teacher means a lot to me.

Plan, plan, plan.

No to the classroom. No to calling my husband. Maybe I should go home and wait for Craig there, or should I go straight to the hospital? I might be bleeding out. That's possible. I've never gone to the emergency room before, but yes, it dawns on me that being home in an empty house is a bad idea if this is as bad as I suspect it might be. I probably *have* to go to the hospital. I don't want help, feel too well for an ambulance, so I guess I'll have to get there on my own.

I walk to my car, breathing slow purposeful breaths, trying to approximate how a regular person looks when she's walking through a parking lot to her car. My shoes are soaking from washing them in the sink, and they make a squelching noise as I near my car. It's July and in the high eighties, and still daylight but not for long. I get three of my swim towels out of the trunk and put them on the driver's seat, try to think clearly, will myself to focus, to think.

Plan, plan, plan.

Program the GPS to the emergency room, I tell myself. OK. Done.

Follow it closely. I remind myself to drive slowly and stay in the right-hand lane so that if I begin to pass out I can pull over and not cause an accident. I don't know what is happening, don't know how much blood is still coming, don't know if something has burst inside me, so I must be careful. And maybe I've stopped bleeding too. That's possible. I can't tell.

I drive and think, If I am dying, if this is how I die, then this is how I die. I am not afraid exactly. For now I just have to drive with precision, thirty-five miles per hour, till I find a parking space near the emergency room of our local hospital and stand at the front desk asking if they will call my husband before I pass out, before I forget his phone number. I want him there next to me, although I am aware of the solitary nature of these moments, even when the people we love are standing right there next to us.

The word *exsanguinate* comes bubbling up into my mind as I drive. Perhaps I am exsanguinating. Bleeding out. It's a magnificent word, *exsanguinate*. *Exsanguination*. Latin, probably. Worth a zillion points in Scrabble.

I decide that I would prefer to die, if I am going to die tonight, in the hospital where people are trained to cope with the mess of death. I don't want to die in my car because it would frighten people on the highway, and Craig would be left with a car full of blood. It would forever be known as "the car my wife died in." No, if I *am* exsanguinating, I will get as close to the hospital as I can, and the second I begin to feel woozy at all, I will get the car over to the shoulder so no one gets hurt.

Something began when I stood up in that classroom, a journey with a hazy destination, my companions for the journey as yet unclear, the potential lessons utterly obscured by the immediacy of the moment. Regardless, I am glad that I wore this pretty dress to class. I am alive, and staying alive requires that I park and make my way, step by step, into the ER, blood pouring down my thighs.

TWO

The Lifted Corner

Ten years before my trip to the emergency room, right after we got married, Craig and I bought an old farmhouse in New Jersey. My tiny black cat, Rosie, moved in and caught the mice that crawled in through the kitchen wall. I fell in love with the pond out back, and with the mallard ducks who nested in the reeds nearby. The chickens next door wandered into our yard and lent our lives a bucolic, permanent air.

When our first spring arrived, I called my mom to tell her I'd found a thousand lilies of the valley beneath our maple tree, just like the ones she'd planted when I was a kid. And Craig, who had been a playful, sweet boyfriend, grew into a playful, sweet husband too, much to my relief.

There were bad times, that first year, mostly my fault. I was jittery. Before Craig there had been a series of bad relationships, and like a puppy from a pound, I flinched at phantoms, so convinced that Craig would cheat or leave. I saw betrayal where it didn't exist.

Money was tight, and I had trouble finding full-time work as a teacher. We fought about joint bank accounts. (I didn't want one.) I was furious at him, poor guy, when the first piece of mail arrived addressed to *Mrs. Craig Lombardi*. Not one piece of my name was on the envelope. I had been subsumed by his identity, or that's what I feared.

One morning as I was leaving for work, I sneezed, and instead of saying "Bless you," Craig said, "Four."

"What?" I asked.

"Four sneezes." He was tying his tie, looking in the hall mirror. "When you sneeze," he said, "you always sneeze four times in a row. I thought you should know." It was such a delicate expression of how closely he was paying attention, an expression of such surprising intimacy. I felt like a thirsty flower, Craig's affection a jar of water soaking my roots.

At night, when I came to bed, even if I had just returned from the bathroom at three in the morning, Craig held up a corner of the blanket for me to get under. Every single time. The tiny gesture hit me so hard, made me so suddenly forgive everyone who had ever hurt me, that I didn't tell him how much I liked it. Craig was afraid of jinxing Notre Dame football, so when they played he wore his lucky underwear. It was for fear of jinxing my good fortune that I never mentioned the lifted corner of the blanket to Craig.

By the end of that first year, as we set up a joint bank account (I kept my own account as well), I began to relax ever so slightly. We settled into a peaceful rhythm of getting to know each other, getting to know the sounds of the house at night, and getting to know ourselves as these new people with titles that belonged still more to our parents than to us. It became clear that we were OK at marriage, that the fears I had brought with me from another life had nothing to do with us. Happiness slowly piled on top of my sorrows and fears and began to submerge them.

THEN I GOT pregnant. When Craig got home from work that day, we sat staring at the pregnancy test. We laughed and then we panicked. "When are the adults coming home?" he asked.

"Seriously."

I was forty-one, and we hadn't planned on having kids. I had no expectations about being a mom, thought it would be OK whether or not we had children. But getting pregnant changed that. The world celebrated when they heard our news. My body hummed. I called my best friend in Chicago. "You're going to be a great mom," she said.

My family was happy too. Mom said she'd come help if I wanted her to. Dad, who was still alive back then, couldn't stop singing songs with words like *baby* in the lyrics. Because his hearing aids were rarely turned on, he sang loudly.

Their joy and my hormones made me deeply invested. I wandered through the baby department at Target looking at tiny outfits the color of candy. Friends advised me what strollers to buy, and people planned parties. It was exciting.

Craig was levelheaded and baby-proofed the house. He took personal days at work so he could join me at doctor appointments, scheduled between my teaching at the local community college. He framed the sonogram that confirmed the baby's heartbeat and put it on his desk. At night I read to him from pregnancy books. When I gave up wine, he gave up beer, and we steered well into the second trimester.

THEN, LIKE THAT, I started to "spot," which sounds harmless, like *spotting* a heron on a tree stump. When I called Dr. G, my gynecologist, he said, "Wait a day. It'll probably stop on its own." But it didn't stop, so Craig took the day off and we went for another sonogram.

I had learned sonogram-technician etiquette by then. When the news was good, she turned the monitor to show us the peanut-sized fetus, and then later, to let us hear the thrum of its heartbeat, like a handful of lightning bugs buzzing in a jelly jar. When we went in this time, though, she wouldn't look at me and said, "I'm not supposed to interpret the sonogram for you. You'll have to speak with your doctor." Well, I knew what that meant, and when the tech left the room, I told Craig that the pregnancy was over.

"We don't know that," he said. He was looking out the window. "Everything's fine," Craig said. "Everything's fine."

We waited under fluorescent lights for Dr. G, who opened the door, looked into the room and into my eyes, and hesitated there on the threshold, his hand behind him still on the doorknob. "You can say it," I said, trying to be kind to him. "It's OK. I already know."

"There's no heartbeat," he said, closing the door behind him as he entered the room with us. Craig, who had been rubbing a single spot on my shoulder, sighed and let his hand drop to his side.

We made an appointment for the next morning for a D&C at the Wayne Surgical Center, behind Trader Joe's. I would be uncomfortable tonight, Dr. G warned. "Get Kotex on your way home." But we didn't stop. It was as though there were menacing clouds on the horizon, so

Craig took me straight home after leaving Dr. G's office, and then kept the car running so he could go back out for supplies. I was beginning to cramp.

"I'm getting into bed," I told Craig, the persistence of what was happening to me physically pushed all thought off. Craig let me out of the car, and as I stood I felt the blood soak the pad I was wearing. "Get me the biggest Kotex you can find, will you?" I supported myself on the car door. "Are you crying?" I asked him. His eyes were red.

"No," he told me, "I just have dust in my eyes." He pulled out of the driveway and left me there.

I WAS GOING to feed Rosie, who was circling around my feet inside the front door, but the cramps were changing to something I couldn't recognize, and I wanted to get to my bed while I still could. The coming night loomed as I walked up the last few steps, hunched over, panting.

I lay in bed on top of spread-out towels, cramps coming in waves, and called my parents. Dad answered the phone. "I'm having a miscarriage," I told him.

"Wait," he said, "I don't have my hearing aids in," and he handed the phone to my mom.

"We just got back from the doctor," I told her, pausing so she could repeat it all for Dad. "We're having a miscarriage. No heartbeat." I could hear my sister, who lived there, in the background say, "Oh no." I wished I was home. I wanted my mom.

As I hung up, the cramps got stronger, unfamiliar, like there was a hallway yawning open inside me. I called Craig's cell and said to his voice mail, "Forget the pads. Just come home."

Then there was the warmth of a lot of blood soaking the pad and maybe the mattress. I couldn't stand up, so I slid onto the floor panting and yelled Craig's name as I inched on hands and knees to the bathroom, the cell phone in my hand in case I needed an ambulance.

Rosie ran to me, first by the bed, then as I crawled down the hallway, and finally into the bathroom. She meowed in my face as I shouted Craig's name, and then she ran back a few feet to wait, and then ran back to me. I thought about childbirth in movies, how people ran around tearing up sheets, and I thought, *Rosie would boil water for me if she could. She would tear up sheets if I needed them.* I remember being grateful to have her as a witness.

I got up from the floor onto the toilet and called Craig's cell phone over and over. Once I yelled, "Hurry home," and once I asked, "Where are you?" and once I just said, "Please." How long had he been gone? As the cramps subsided, I called Dr. G, who said, "We can get you an ambulance if you want, but it sounds like you are miscarrying right now. By the time we get you here, it'll be over. Do you want to be home for this or in the hospital?"

There was a lot of blood. "Am I dying?" I asked.

"No," he said, "You're going to be all right. It just feels like you're dying. Your body is doing what it's supposed to do, expelling the dead tissue." He gave me his home and cell numbers, which I wrote in eyeliner on the back of an ESPN magazine that was next to the toilet. Once I knew I'd survive, I wanted to be home in our bed when it was all over.

I gave in to my body. When it was still, I pet Rosie, and when the waves resurfaced, I shouted for Craig. I called him on the phone one last time and said, "It's happening right now."

Finally, the inside of my body from up under my ribcage down to the bottom of my spine heaved and shuddered, and out slipped something, that when I looked in the toilet, looked like a crescent moon carved from soft opal. My body relaxed.

I cleaned the bathroom and myself, then went back to bed. (A decade later I would find myself wiping up another bathroom floor.) Rosie climbed onto the pillow next to my head. I half realized, as I drifted off, that I must have been in labor.

By the time Craig rustled in with plastic grocery bags full of supplies, the room was dark. "How long have you been gone?" I asked.

"I don't know, half an hour?"

He sat on the bed. "I think it's over," I said, sleepy, sorrow creeping into the space left by the retreating fear. "I think I had the miscarriage just now."

"I got your messages," he said, lying down on the bed and petting my hair. "I forgot to turn on my phone. You called seventeen times. I listened to the first one in the driveway and then just came up." He lay there and listened to all of the messages then. He saved them too, for a while, before finally deleting them. He said they made his heart race.

I THOUGHT THAT when something awful happened, I'd lie in bed unable to move forever. But it wasn't like that. "I'm cold," I said, so Craig pulled the blankets up, "and Rosie needs food."

Later Craig said, "I found some old videos I made of an *Odd Couple* marathon. Let's have ice cream for dinner and watch *The Odd Couple*. How does that sound?"

"Sure," I said, taking one of the plastic bags he'd

brought home with him into the bathroom. "That sounds fine."

He brought me his Notre Dame ski cap. "To keep you warm." We watched *The Odd Couple* and ate bowls of chocolate ice cream, and we laughed, just like that. I didn't expect to laugh or for the ice cream to taste good, but it did.

"I'm sleepy," I said, "but leave the tape on, OK?" I wanted to listen to Oscar and Felix argue, wanted to hear the 1970s laugh track as I fell asleep.

WE WENT FOR the D&C in the morning. They put me on a table, my arms strapped out in a cross, and clipped a plastic hose to my nostrils. The gas smelled bitter. I winced and then nothingness. At home, later, I watched five videotapes of *The Odd Couple* and ate ice cream for dinner again. Craig put Rosie's dish by the bed so that she'd eat.

By the next morning I was sick of *The Odd Couple*, sick of the ice cream, sick of bed. My sister was coming to visit, so I made a pot of rosemary stew like Mom used to make. There was old snow on the ground. I wanted meat and carrots and rosemary, wanted to fill up my belly with something warm and healing.

By the time my sister arrived, the house was steamy from the cooking stew. I had the ski cap on, would keep it on all weekend. My sister made the calls that had to be made. I couldn't do it, wasn't ready to tell people the bad news over and over and then console them.

WE GOT PREGNANT twice again, but kept those to ourselves, never made the mistake of telling people, which made subsequent losses easier on us, if more isolated.

These things happen, we told ourselves. I got full-time work as a university lecturer, teaching writing. We reminded ourselves of how we were lucky, how we had each other, and this old house, with its pond, where the mallards returned every spring to nest and mate. And then, well, life moved on. And all of that was a distant memory years later when I visited the emergency room that summer night.

THREE

Dilation and Curettage

Dilation and curettage (D&C) is a procedure to remove tissue from inside your uterus. Doctors perform dilation and curettage to diagnose and treat certain uterine conditions—such as heavy bleeding—or to clear the uterine lining after a miscarriage or abortion.

In a dilation and curettage . . . your doctor uses small instruments or a medication to open (dilate) your cervix—the lower, narrow part of your uterus. Your doctor then uses a surgical instrument called a curette to remove uterine tissue. Curettes used in a D&C can be sharp or use suction.

—MayoClinic.org

After all that blood and my trip to the emergency room, I'm home, and other than being shaken, I'm OK. The bleeding has slowed back down from alarming to heavy, and I decide I can return to night two of my writing class.

The day after that is my appointment with my gynecologist. I tell him what happened, that I had this sudden and alarming amount of blood, went to the ER, the bleeding subsided, and now what? The doctor tells me that we should do a D&C to try and figure out why there is so much blood, so about three days after the ER visit, I'm back at the same dreary place I went years ago, after the earlier miscarriages, at the Wayne Surgical Center behind Trader Joe's on Hamburg Turnpike. (Could anything be more depressing?)

Dilation is the widening of the cervix. *Curettage* is the scraping out of the effluvia in the uterus. Words are sometimes pretty, sometimes descriptive, sometimes explanatory, but not usually all three. *Curettage* is a prettier word than *scraping*, but *scraping* is more accurate, more graphic, more frank.

Paperwork and health insurance are the bureaucracy of my illness, whatever this illness turns out to be. How many times must I tell these strangers my birthdate? With all the computers buzzing around us, don't they know who I am? Again and again they ask for my date of birth. It feels so impersonal for such a vulnerable moment: "Date of birth?" They don't even look up from their glowing screens, their clipboards, and if anyone smiles at me in the outer office, they don't smile all the way to their eyes.

It feels dystopian, another way for them to demonstrate how little they know or care about me, to remind me that I am one of a long line of women lining up here today to be gowned, splayed on a table, and scraped clean, like mackerel.

I think of Grandma Hastings, whose interest in biology, chemistry, and physics made her dream of becoming a doctor. That was frowned upon for women of her era, but she studied biology at Sophie Newcomb anyway and became a lab technician at Charity Hospital in New Orleans. She was proud, my mother told me, that she was one of the few lab techs who could quickly identify typhoid from a slide. So I think of her and of how I was allowed to sleep in her bed with her when I was five. I wish I could infuse the clinicians at Wayne Surgical Center with a combination of her medical savvy and her deep love for me.

But it doesn't work. This is a different time and place, and I remain aware that these people don't want to get sued because of operating on the wrong person, so they check and double-check my date of birth. It's clear that I am both a patient deserving of gentle care and a problem who must be managed correctly to take up the right amount of allotted time. Oh, I am also a potential litigant. They are likely afraid that I will sue them, and I am afraid that they might think of me as only a birth date, or an annoyance, and will further injure this one body of mine. We are foes in some fundamental way that I find inescapable while I frantically try to think of a way to make them care about me as they would for a friend or family member.

Craig has taken the day off from work to be with me, but we're pulled apart after the paperwork—another inexplicable cruelty—and I find myself in a gown and on a gurney in a chilly, curtained-off room. They have put a thin yellow blanket over my legs, and I'm willing myself to stay calm, to breathe, to think about happy things like my garden and the ancient but failing pear tree in our backyard. I have a shower cap over my hair and a needle in the crook of my arm attached to a hose and a bottle, the bottle hanging on a metal coatrack-looking thing. I'm cold. And I'm bleeding, of course.

The fifth or sixth nurse enters my curtained area. She's wearing scrubs and carrying a clipboard. She is annoyed by something, I can tell, something outside of me, but still, her annoyance is with her in my tiny, curtained-off, freezing "room." I take a deep breath.

"Date of birth?" she says, not looking up. She's clicking her pen. *Click click click*. She wants to punch someone. That's what it feels like, and I'm sure that if I knew the details, I'd be on her side, but since I've been asked my date of birth at least five times already, I'm annoyed, and have to will myself not to sigh or roll my eyes as I recite my date of birth . . . again.

"Do you know what you are here for today?" She hasn't looked up yet. *Click click click*.

"A D and C," I say, wanting her to look at me. "Dilation and curettage." I want her to see that I am smart. "With a hysteroscopy," I add. I am no dummy. It's a way of asserting my humanness to know big words, to understand what is happening to me. I try to convey all that to this stranger as I sit here, without underwear on, bleeding all over the gurney, ashamed.

"Have you had any prior surgeries?" she asks, sighing. Poor thing, she's probably had to ask this question a dozen times this morning alone. She's bored, in addition to seeming angry. *Hurry up*, I feel her saying to me with her mind.

"I've had three miscarriages, and I think only one required a D and C afterward."

"So is this your second surgery?"

I'm not sure. I may have had another D&C in there somewhere. I'm getting confused and wish that Craig was with me. In our house, he is the one who is in charge of numbers, and I am in charge of words. But he is back in the waiting room.

She taps her pen against her clipboard. What does it matter how many surgeries I've had?

"How many children do you have?" she asks. *Tap tap tap*.

I wish she'd leave me alone. "None," I say, and I feel my jaw tighten as I try to say it the way a normal person would say it, as though I'm just answering a simple question.

"Oh dear," she says, letting her pen and clipboard fall in front of her stomach. All of a freaking sudden she's looking at me. Like really looking. "How awful." Her eyes become puddles. Then so do mine. I could kill her. She's crying and has gone from not seeing me at all to seeing way too much of me, and there is no curtain for me to draw between us. The pity in her eyes and all the sorrow of the gone-by years wash over me like a drowning wave, pulling the garden and the woods and the deep breathing out of reach. I am fine, I tell myself, I am fine. But all of the picturing of Craig's smiling blue eyes is erased, so that when they wheel me in for surgery,

I'm upset, rattled, the until-now-submerged sorrow bobbing to the surface.

Fuckers.

WHEN THE D&C is over, Craig and I go home to await the pathology report to find out what is happening to my body. It takes some time, a week maybe, and all that week while we await results, the only pain I feel is from where some orderly ripped the tape off my arm to take out the IV needle.

In fact, even months later, after everything unfolds, I will still have a scar from where the adhesive lifted off the delicate skin inside the crook of my elbow. It will be the only scar I'll ever see from this, or from anything that is about to happen to me, and provides some sort of tangible evidence that anything ever happened to me at all.

FOUR

The Feral Cat
and the French Fries

Feral cat: A feral cat is a cat who has either never had any contact with humans or her contact with humans has diminished over time. She's fearful of people and survives on her own outdoors.

—Alleycat.org

For years now, I've been dancing a dance with a feral cat, wiry and ugly, skinny as a fist, his face striped right down the middle, one half black, the other orange. He is my little unhoused ghost.

I figure it's a "he" because he and Zonker, our male cat, howl at one another over the summer nights, the peepers in the background singing harmony. Other nights he yowls all alone by the compost bin. I want to go to him, but if I make a sound, if I disturb the air currents between us, he can feel it in his whiskers, and vanishes.

After Rosie died, we got two badger-sized cats from the pound, part Maine coon, enormous all by themselves and overfed on top of that. They're brother and sister, and identical except that Zonker (the male) has only one good eye. Craig chose Zonker's name and I named Crinkle (the female). When they lie on top of me in bed (which I encourage them to do), I can hardly breathe under the weight of them.

He was gone once for almost a year, the feral cat. I fretted, always looking, assuming his death, I hoped not from starvation, which seemed a protracted and awful way to die. But then I saw him under the rhododendron, plump almost, and I was filled with such joy. I leaned against the kitchen door, my arms folded, beaming, knowing that any noise would make him run down to the pond and then on into the woods near the abbey. Do the monks feed him there? I hope he has somewhere to go where he can rely on someone.

WE HAVE A neighbor, a woman with gray hair to her waist. She rescues roosters, which makes her a bad neighbor but a decent human being. She talks and talks, this neighbor, as though no one has ever listened to her before, and sometimes I just have to walk away from her down her long driveway with her still talking at my back, telling me over and over again her same stories of loss. "How do you make friends?" she asked me once. How *do* you make friends?

In summer when we have our windows open, I can hear her encouraging her hens. "Now Lucy," I'll hear her say, "I've told you a hundred times not to step in the water dish."

ONE DAY DURING one of my mother's regular visits to our farmhouse in New Jersey, we were, as was our habit, sitting in the sunroom around five, drinking gin and looking out at the wildlife. There were groundhogs and wild turkeys, an occasional chicken from next door came clucking through the lilacs scratching for grubs. We kept an eye out for hummingbirds in the bee balm, and for the mallard family that returns every spring to nest by Domer Pond.

We had eaten lunch that day at a diner and, back at home, had thrown our leftover french fries in the grass to see if we might attract a crow or, better yet, a turkey vulture, but nothing happened. We sat and drank, talking intermittently about things like my father's death (which came in 2013 after all of the miscarriages were over and we'd given up on kids) or the *Times Book Review*, or whatever came to mind, when all of a sudden there was the feral cat out in the longish grass, all angles, thin as a reed. He paused, and lifted his head up, his ears like antennae. Sniffing the air, he lowered his head and began gobbling the french fries, darting glances to his side like a prisoner guarding his meal. We put our martini glasses down and leaned toward him, drawn by the enormity of his hunger. When did he eat last? How long can a cat go without eating? How close to death must a cat be to eat potatoes?

THAT AFTERNOON WITH Mom a few years ago, there was the cat on the lawn. The mallards by the pond were there too, so it must have been late summer, and there was a mole I knew had been in the yard by the hill of grass it had pushed up. Our enormous cats were nearby, asleep on the futon. The roosters were crowing their lungs out next door, and I could imagine my long-haired neighbor, the one with all the rescued roosters, whispering to no one, unspooling her loneliness onto her empty driveway, while this fist of a feral cat ate potatoes in the grass to keep himself alive. All of us, the cats, the mallards, the mole, the neighbor, my mother—if push came to shove, every one of us would eat the french fries out of the grass, right?

Now that I am sick I reach back to that day with Mom often. I lie in the dark, crushed in our warm bed by pillows and Craig and the cats, all so tender, all so safe and fat. I put food out on the porch for the feral cat because I must be able to tell myself that I reached out to the starving cat. I can't do nothing. And so the food goes out, as much for me as for him.

FIVE

Waving to Mom through the Hospital Window

When I was three or four years old, I had two minor traumas. The first was that we moved to a big house in the woods out on Teatown Road in Croton from a tiny one on Quaker Bridge, where my sister and I had shared a room so tiny that our beds touched. On Teatown Road I slept in my own bedroom, which was supposed to be a step up in the world. I guess I let my profound loneliness be known, because soon enough I was sharing my sister's room again, a port in the storm of that cavernous house.

The second trauma was that Mom, my full-time companion at that age, went into the hospital because she was in tremendous pain. The doctors knew it was something to do with her kidneys, but they simply could not figure out what it was.

I was bereft without her. "Where is she?" I asked over and over again, and "When is she coming home?"

I remember my poor father taking me to the Red Door Nursery School, and I can still see my white-knuckled fingers clutching at the car seat as he pulled me from the car. "I have to go to work," he begged over my screams.

Children weren't allowed in the hospital then, but as the youngest of four, I know I, for one, needed to see my mom, needed to be reassured that she was still alive, that she was coming back home one day.

Dad put us all in the car one evening, and we drove to a grassy slope outside Phelps Memorial Hospital (where I was born, and where, one day, Grandma Hastings would die). He must have arranged things with Mom because when Dad pointed at a window a few stories up, there was Mom! She waved and called down, and I waved back with all my might, as though it might bring her home or leave me there. Again, Poor Dad. I guess he had to take us home and give us dinner, but all I remember is the feeling of my hand waving, the smell of the grass, the thought that if I waved hard enough I might get to be held by her, I might fly up to reach her.

MUCH LATER, IN my forties, I asked Mom about her time in the hospital. "Oh, they thought it was kidney stones, but it turned out I had some kind of congenital malformation that didn't surface until then, however old I was, thirty or something. They fixed it surgically and I was absolutely fine, if you recall." I didn't, of course. "My mother," she went on, "forever the scientist, I remember her saying when it was all over, 'Annie, the kidneys are so difficult to reach you know, because they're protected by a thick covering of fat. I imagine those doctors had to put you on your side for that operation and move your intestines out of the way so that they could really take a look at things.' I have no idea if they had to do that or not, but ever since I've pictured myself lying on that gurney with my intestines sitting on the table next to me like a chain of breakfast sausages."

SIX

Fireflies and Lightning Bugs

With the D&C over and the pathology results from it coming soon, I see now that I've been getting ill very gradually, and probably should have realized earlier that something serious was brewing. I had been bleeding pretty heavily for about five months before I ended up in the emergency room. I had a few days here and there with no blood, but for the most part, I was a mess, day in and day out, for those five months.

I justified not doing anything about it because, well, maybe it was just perimenopause. Your body changes in your fifties. Plus I had already spent so much time with my gynecologist around all of the miscarriages, that I sort of shied away from going back. I didn't want a bunch of tests, didn't want to be poked and prodded and then told what I already assumed would be the boring explanation, "Well, you're in your fifties now, so this is natural." I thought I'd get through it on my own.

But over those five months, I became increasingly isolated. There wasn't anything specific to report to friends, but when the flow was especially heavy, I begged off meeting friends, never telling them why. What was there to say? I just wanted to be home, to be near a bathroom, near a change of clothes. I didn't tell anyone about it because there wasn't anything real to say. You can't blurt out that you're bleeding a lot. Seems intimate and vague and probably gross, and I figured everyone else was bleeding a lot too.

While I thought that the D&C would stop the bleeding, sadly it hasn't, so whatever was wrong with me before the D&C is still wrong, and I hope that the pathologist's results will be decisive, giving me something tangible to tell people, because again, even though I've been to the emergency room now, there's still nothing to say.

I'M AWARE, HOWEVER, that by not telling anyone, this whole amorphous situation is turning into a secret that I never meant to keep. From the outside I guess it just looks like I'm blowing people off, canceling plans, acting distant. Plus I'm pretty exhausted from being unwell, and I get the feeling that I am not thinking in a crisp manner. Trying to figure out who to tell and how to bring it up is too much to cope with.

I imagine saying to my neighbor, "So now that our Pilates class is over, I just wanted to tell you that I've been bleeding like crazy for like forEVER." Just kidding. I don't even really know what Pilates is.

Being frank has its difficulties, but I don't want to be all hushed or melodramatic either. I don't feel hushed and melodramatic about this, whatever *this* is. The thing is, though, that I've canceled so many plans without explanation that I've become one of *those* friends. Yes, I still leave home, but less and less frequently. By now I've had so many times when I've bled through my clothes that I am forever considering how far away from home is too far, and how many minutes of hanging out is too many minutes, and this was all before going to the ER and having a D&C. Many months prior I had already stopped sitting on anyone's furniture for fear of ruining it.

As I AWAIT the results from pathology, it's August and the teaching job that I thought I had for September has fallen through. I don't even know if I'll be able to teach, but this feels bad. I'm worried about money, without really having the mental bandwidth to worry effectively (whatever effective worry looks like). Ashamed, conflicted, and physically unwell, I apply for unemployment, something I've never done before, but I know I won't be able to get work with school about to get underway, and I want to be able to pay my share of the mortgage. It's difficult to get unemployment and it keeps me busy for a day or two filling out all the paperwork, making the requisite phone calls, while I wait to hear from my doctor about what's next. When I learn that I will receive unemployment, I feel as though I've won the lottery. I won't have to borrow money or use up my savings while doctors determine what's happening with all of this blood.

ON ONE OF the waiting days, I take my book out to a chair on the lawn to sit in the sun and read, although I end up sitting there with my eyes closed, the sun warming me. It dawns on me that if I am walking around pretending that everything's fine, there might be a lot of other people who are also pretending that everything's fine.

I think of my grandmother's calendar, the tiny one I found in a box in the attic recently. It hung on her bedroom wall the year she lived with us before she died. She seemed so well, as I sat with her in her bedroom every day and watched Julia Child on her black-and-white TV. Almost fifty years later, I look at that Norcross calendar and see Grandma's tiny notes to herself. Written in ballpoint pen on the back of January 1969: *Snow kept dr away—lowest energy—couldn't finish writing letters.* I was five. How could I have known? On the back of February, she wrote simply: *holding my own.*

Maybe everyone is made up of two rivers, the part on the surface that the sun hits, and the cool part that runs over the river rocks in the shadows that no one can see.

The underside of my own river is likely the same as the underside of everyone else's, and the fact that my physical frailty connects me to Grandma Hastings and probably to everyone else is a revelation, makes me feel cozy, makes the world shimmer, helps me begin to relax about telling people.

I sit in a chair on our lawn holding my unread book in my lap, thinking how *not* alone I probably am. Being sick makes me less alone than I've ever been, when I look at it like that.

We are all of us separated from one another in countless ways. Half the country says "lightning bug" while the other half says "firefly," for just one very small example. What a shock to realize that illness and brokenness are practically universal, while wholeness is the ephemeral state, longed for precisely because it's attained only momentarily, if at all.

Being unwell connects me to most of the people who say firefly and most of the people who say lightning bug. For this one moment, I'm OK, and maybe I don't need to go out of my way to tell people what's happening. Those who need to, know already, and when there is something to tell, I'll know what to do.

SEVEN

The Dove on the Door

At eighty, in frail health, Grandma Hastings came to live with us in my childhood home in Croton-on-Hudson in Westchester County, New York. My maternal grandfather had died years before—I never even met him—and she could no longer live on her own. She wore a kind of back brace that she called a corset, and she had a heart problem, not that I understood any of that when she moved into our wildly busy house. Dad was an announcer on WQXR, the classical music radio station of the *New York Times* in New York City. Mom was making art. There were four of us kids under fifteen, plus three snakes in terrariums in my oldest brother's room, and six cats, two dogs, and thirteen chickens, all of whom lived outside. Oh, and my sister had a rabbit named Hasty Two. (Hasty One had died the year before, but *Hasty* was such a good name for a rabbit that she had to use the name again).

The geographic road that led Grandma to our home in Westchester started in New Orleans, went through

Washington Square Park in New York City when she married my grandfather, then to Washington, DC, when her husband got a job as speechwriter for President Herbert Hoover, then back to New York City, and when her husband had spent what he'd made and then some on booze and other women, they moved to Ridgewood, New Jersey, where this former New Orleans socialite and Queen of Rex 1911 worked as a substitute teacher and took in boarders to make ends meet.

When she moved into our house, decades after my grandfather had died, the first thing she did (after she'd unpacked her entire lifetime into one room on the ground floor of her daughter's house) was to thumbtack a Christmas card of a dove holding an olive branch in its beak to her bedroom door.

She gathered us kids together and said in her still-lovely uptown New Orleans accent, "This," she motioned to her door and to her room beyond, "this is the room of peace."

And so it was.

I was the youngest, and as such, was chased everywhere I went for the first ten years of my life. I knew that if I could make it to Grandma's room, I would be safe. No one dared to enter there with malice in their hearts. There was no tickling allowed, no yelling or guffawing.

She was the oldest, and she and I formed the alpha and omega, my life beginning, hers drawing to an end very soon. She had one year with us, and because we both found ourselves on the margins of this frenetic, lively, ebullient family, we took solace in one another. I could be quiet and safe in her room with her. She could be needed.

EIGHT

Plausible Eternity

I like nature, and that when I die the earthworms will eat me up and use me the same way they use the dead maple leaves and the fallen pine needles. I am more than just OK with that. I *love* that. It's a kind of plausible eternity.

Some people call me spiritual, which troubles me. I don't like labels, and *spiritual* feels as if it's a box people want to put me in when they see that I'm not religious. They can't conceive of people who don't believe in God in a particular way. But maybe *spiritual* to them is just shorthand for them noticing how much I like the world.

I'm a little bit prickly about this stuff. It's private and complicated, and I figure that the way every person worships or doesn't worship is, and also that there are as many different ways of being an atheist as there are of being a Christian, a Jew, or a Muslim. It's not like I can change what I believe anyway. Isn't that what belief is?

Do we really believe something if we can be bullied out of believing it?

Sometimes I think people call me spiritual because it's their way of allowing me into their club, and that feels all right to me, and not like judgment but more like sweetness, although I'm not a big fan of clubs. I am difficult in this way, wanting everything and nothing at once, wanting to be both at the party and in the attic above the party, just listening in. Craig just wants to be at the party. He is a flat line and I am a roller coaster, and over the years we exert some gravitational force that pulls him more toward roller coaster and me more toward flat line. Still, I don't think of the word *spiritual* when I think of myself. It's a word people use to help them understand what is hard to understand about me, I guess.

As I AWAIT the results of the post-ER D&C, the one or two people who know I'm sick want to pray for me, not like I'm on my deathbed but just the casual, "I'll keep you in my prayers" kind of thing. I am not an angry atheist like my father was (he was angry about religion for reasons that I think made sense) or an angry atheist like one of my siblings (who is angry about religion because our father was angry about it, although, to be fair, most people's beliefs are hereditary, acquired like hand-me-downs). I don't hate religion. If someone wants to pray for me, it's OK with me. My father, on the other hand, would have hated that. He made sure the people at the nursing home didn't send anyone, a priest or a rabbi, to bother him. To Dad, someone praying for him felt like a trap, which I could also see. (And yes, it is sometimes exhausting seeing both sides of everything.)

My father became an atheist because he bridled under his childhood household's Orthodox Judaism. I didn't grow up in that kind of household, though. I told him my thoughts on the subject toward the end of his life, when he was in the nursing home. We'd sit on the porch there and I'd read poetry to him, and we would chat, or not even that sometimes. By the end even sitting up was difficult for him, and so sometimes sitting next to one another in silence was what we did. "I'm not as angry about religion as you are," I told him, warming his hands.

"You were always smarter than I was," he said, his eyes closed, his face still, the clouds hanging above us in the sky. That is a nice thing for a dying father to tell his daughter. By then, Dad had so little strength that I felt I could trust that he was his essential self, unmediated. I

could believe that he meant what he was saying because
he no longer had the energy or cunning to lie or be polite.
He died well in that way, with all of the kind things he
had stored up said aloud.

I CAN FEEL myself being changed by this illness. Time
passes differently as I wait to find out what is wrong
with me, and my thoughts slow down too, and deepen.
I notice things more carefully—the angle of the twigs
protruding from the birdhouse hanging in the lilacs, the
sound of Zonker's deep breathing when he sleeps, the
way the blood is rustling around in my veins, and the
way I am poised for whatever train is coming down the
tracks toward me. Time creeps to a standstill, and we all
pause and breathe: me, the starlings making a nest in the
gutter, the blood in my body, waiting for the air currents
to shift before we decide what to do next. I am not sure,
but I think this is what some people mean by *God*, this
stillness inside an approaching hurricane.

NINE

The Brightness of the Middle

My father died a slow death, and because of that I want a quick one. I want to grow old too, which I guess is at odds with wanting a quick death. To grow old is, by definition almost, to consign oneself to a slow, incremental death. Death by old age starts with a sore knee and digestive discomfort and proceeds from there, an inch at a time. But I would like to both grow old *and* die quickly. There, I said it. I want it all.

While my father also wanted a fast death, it turns out that it's not the kind of thing a person can pull off, not the kind of thing we're in control of, like they try to make you think it is in movies. He spent eight months in a nursing home trying to die. "Take me off my meds," he told us, and we did with no result. Every day he'd say, in one way or another, that he was ready, that he wanted to die, that he was miserable over being alive.

"You know, Dad," I said to him one day, "if you

really want to die, you still have control over what you eat. You could stop eating, stop drinking."

He thought for a minute, then said, "But I love to eat," so we brought him bags of KitKats and unwrapped them three at a time. At least there was that.

My father had a great life, but he didn't get the death he wanted. Instead, he had strangers leaning him up against the cold tile walls of the nursing home shower to clean him after he went to the bathroom. There was a machine they used, a Hoyer lift, to haul his curving bones out of bed every morning—his fingers curving up, his toes curving down, his neck curving to the side like he was a wet leaf, its drying edges curling in as it lay on the windowsill.

AFTER HE DIED, my mom, my sister, and I fantasized about good ways to go. I said I'd like to be crossing Fifth Avenue and have a bus come out of nowhere and just run me down. My sister said, "Well, you better hope you don't get dragged."

"Right."

On a train the winter after Dad died, my mother looked down over the edge of a trestle bridge. "If you fell from up here onto the ice down there, you'd probably die instantly," she said, "and if not instantly, then you'd freeze or drown."

"But freezing to death takes a long time," my sister said, "and what if you don't break your neck? Then you're just lying on the ice, suffering." It's the suffering we want to avoid, and the utter dependence on people, often strangers.

"Teddy Roosevelt died in his sleep," I said. I'd been rewatching the Roosevelt documentary on PBS.

"Who did?" my mother asked. I had to shout at her now that she was losing her hearing.

"TEDDY ROOSEVELT!"

"Oh."

"His hands were folded across his chest in the morning like everything was fine." I didn't exactly shout this time.

"How great. He just woke up dead," Mom said. It did sound great. "Where can I sign up to die like Teddy Roosevelt?"

People say that death is the great leveler, and yes, kings and all of us regular serf types face it. Even the greedy die. Even the famous. What precedes death is also pretty universal. Final illnesses are often messy and humiliating, confusing and frightening. Everyone wants to die with dignity, but almost no one does, except apparently, for Teddy Roosevelt, who some might call a show-off, he died so peacefully.

In his poem "I Have Good News," the poet Tony Hoagland wrote: "The dark ending does not cancel out / the brightness of the middle," or so I remind myself. If I can't control the ending, then at least I can try to have a bright middle.

STILL, MY MOTHER has figured out a few things. When Dad got sick, they moved their bedroom downstairs into Grandma Hastings' old room. There is a big rock outside of Mom's bedroom window there, with a bowl-like indentation in it that fills up with water when it rains. When I visit her, I sometimes catch her topping off the water in the puddle with a little watering can. "If I keep my puddle full, I can watch the birds hopping in it all day long." She has instructed me that if she is ever out of it like Dad was, she wants to be able to see her puddle full of birds, that she can be happy as long as she can see them.

My husband has asked that if he ends up incapacitated, he'd like me to keep a steady stream of winning Notre Dame football games on TV for him. He's set up a shelf of recordings of the games he wants to watch, going all the way back to the 1980s.

Maybe this is the way to cope with illness and dying. If Mom has to go eventually, a point which I very grudgingly concede, we can at least keep her puddle full of water and hopping birds within sight of her bedroom window. For Dad, it was the endless KitKat bars, melted chocolate on his fingertips. And for Craig it will be watching football games where he can be surprised every time Notre Dame scores the winning touchdown, even if he's seen the game a thousand times. If we can't control how and when we die, maybe we can fill the time leading up to our deaths with the joy of carbohydrates, hopping birds, and touchdowns, over and over and over.

TEN

Hemangioma

hemangioma (hē,manjē'ōmə): a benign tumor of blood vessels, often forming a red birthmark
—ArchivesofPathology.org

Tissues from my D&C are sent to the pathologist, who gives me a diagnosis: I have a uterine hemangioma, which is pretty much a birthmark on my uterus. A birthmark on my uterus. And me, never able to have children. All those miscarriages, so distant now that it's sometimes like they happened to someone else, like I read the story somewhere.

I named one, the miscarriage that happened in my second trimester. Cole. I named him Cole although I never told anyone that before just now. This was after the doctor let us listen to his heartbeat.

Anyway.

Also according to the Archives of Pathology website, a uterine hemangioma "is a rare benign tumor" that presents either as a pregnancy-related complication or around excessively heavy menstrual bleeding. It's rare too, with only fifty cases diagnosed in the United States.

ELEVEN

Diagnosis

A diagnosis can be a powerful tool. I find that having a name for my conglomeration of symptoms is galvanizing. I can look up symptoms, weigh and consider the choices at hand, see how others have coped. Nothing essential changes with a diagnosis. It's not a cure, yet on some basic level having a diagnosis also changes absolutely everything. All of my anticipation, the worry about worst-case scenarios, has vanished. There are steps I can take, after all, to mitigate or even fix a uterine hemangioma.

MY DIAGNOSIS REMINDS me of when my father, after years of incrementally failing health, was finally diagnosed with multiple system atrophy (MSA), which shares many of the symptoms of Parkinson's, so the diagnosis explained Dad's chronically cold hands as well as his vision problems. (He was probably suffering from something called ocular palsies.) MSA also accounted for his falling (due to his diminished postural reflexes, a Parkinsonian thing), as well as his fainting (due to orthostatic hypotension). One of the symptoms of MSA can be agitated sleep due to acting out one's dreams. This explained why he had hit Mom in his sleep. The fractured drawing of a clock he'd made at the neurologist's office now gave us a window into how he was struggling to perceive the world, and that he was seeing a clock in a way that no longer made sense to the rest of us yet still meant "clock" to him. It was an elegant expression of his visuospatial dysfunction. And his walking one step behind us, it turned out, was not him trying to be annoying. No, it was his way of adapting to the Parkinsonian difficulty of initiating one's own movement. He was instinctively positioning himself to watch my feet to help him walk. My impatience with him fell away after the diagnosis.

Now that I had my diagnosis, a certain calm descended. I had something real, not imagined, and it was rare. It might even account for my many miscarriages over the years.

TWELVE

The Plan

TYPES OF HYSTERECTOMY

Depending on your condition, your surgeon will remove some or all of your uterus and possibly additional parts of your reproductive system.

- *Total Hysterectomy:* The surgeon removes your uterus and your cervix, but not your ovaries. Total hysterectomy is the most common type of hysterectomy.
- *Hysterectomy with Oophorectomy:* The surgeon removes your uterus, one or both of your ovaries, and sometimes your fallopian tubes.
- *Radical Hysterectomy:* The surgeon removes your uterus, cervix, the top portion of your vagina, most of the tissue that surrounds the cervix, and sometimes the pelvic lymph nodes.
- *Supracervical Hysterectomy:* The surgeon removes the body of your uterus, but leaves your cervix intact. Supracervical hysterectomy can treat noncancerous conditions like fibroids or endometriosis.

—Stanfordhealthcare.org

I am in the same doctor's office now that I was in a few years ago for all three miscarriages. But today it is Dr. G's colleague, Dr. S, who is my doctor. Dr. S has a cadence to his voice that reminds me of my father's mother, Grandma Moss. I did not have a close relationship with her the way that I did with Grandma Hastings (my mother's mother), but still, his resemblance to Grandma Moss is enough to make him feel like family. He is gray, tiny, and slim, and peeks out over his little glasses at me.

I've done my own research on uterine hemangiomas and have reached my own decision about treatment, but I want to hear what Dr. S has decided first, to see if we've come to the same conclusion. We have, which is reassuring.

1. *Hysterectomy (Remove the Uterus)*: That's a no-brainer. She's got to go. We could try other things, like ablation, but that can be painful and ineffective. I'm almost past childbearing physically (and way past childbearing emotionally), and it's time to stop the madness.

2. *Salpingectomy (Remove the Fallopian Tubes)*: We don't have to remove these. They aren't diseased, but it looks like people without their fallopian tubes are slightly less likely to develop ovarian cancer.

So if he can reach them easily when he's getting my uterus, he'll get both fallopian tubes as well. This is called prophylactic removal because we'd be removing them before they have to go, in a bid to prevent further disease.

3. *Leave the Ovaries*: There's no sign of disease there, and they produce hormones that I'll need to get me through menopause when this is all over. I'd rather avoid synthetic hormone replacement if possible, and statistics show that keeping one's ovaries leads to a slightly longer life expectancy, so that's an easy choice. Yup. Keeping the ovaries. (On a side note, though, I do like the name of the surgery to remove the ovaries: *oophorectomy*. As a name, it's a thousand times better than *hysterectomy*, but beggars can't be choosers.)

DR. S AND I agree that he'll go in vaginally, so he won't be cutting through the abdominal muscles, which should mean that I'll have a short recovery time of a week or so. "But I won't know till I get in there," Dr. S says, blinking at me over his glasses, a softness in his eyes. I can see he knows sorrow, that he's been through things, and I like that. He seems kind. He is not cocky. This is a good mix for my frazzled, empty veins. "However, if I go in vaginally and there are problems, I'll have to decide right then and there if I need to go in through your abdomen, so be prepared."

I don't know how to prepare for that. I say, "OK," because that's what you say.

I see Grandma Moss in Dr. S's face, hear her in his voice, and it makes me feel like he'll do his best for me. That grandmother, who has been dead for decades, escaped the pogroms with her mother. She worked in sweatshops in New York City sewing sequins onto dresses and fake fruit onto hats. I look at my doctor and I see Grandma Moss, and I think, *All right. She knew her share of sorrow too.*

THIRTEEN

Abandon Hope

Each year approximately 600,000 hysterectomies are performed in the United States, i.e. a little more than one uterus for every minute of the year. . . . This incredible number of surgeries means that approximately one third of American women will have had a hysterectomy by the age of 60.

—Brighamandwomens.org

The surgery I am going to get then is a total hysterectomy, which is a little bit misleading because they aren't taking my ovaries. Taking my ovaries sounds "total" to me, but they are leaving those and removing my fallopian tubes if they can. I remind myself that's called a total hysterectomy with a salpingectomy. They should find another name for this operation. The fact that the uterus is equated with hysteria makes me feel like we're living in Salem, during the witch trials. Surely we could call this something that matches what's actually being done, like uterus-removal surgery. I can't think of anything better at the moment, but the word *hysterectomy* is outdated, and adds insult to injury. What the hell?

A hysterectomy is not a big deal medically. I am not dying, not critically ill, and this is a common surgery. We don't talk about it much, but millions of women in the US have had hysterectomies. So my chances of survival and total recovery are pretty close to 100 percent, and while it's a big deal to have any kind of surgery, I remind myself to keep things in perspective. It's not the hugest deal on earth. Unless, of course, something goes wrong.

Plus it will be a relief to have the bleeding stop, and to put—*Once and For All*—the obsessions with fertility to rest. It will be a good thing to close a door, to abandon all hope of biological children.

I GO HOME after meeting with Dr. S and wait, fretful and uneasy despite my pep talk to myself, waiting now to find out the date of my surgery. I begin getting ready without exactly doing anything yet. I can't think of anything to do, or rather, there is so much to do (and almost none of it matters) that it's hard to figure out where to begin.

As excited as I am to get it over with, I still have to face surgery itself, and feel like a person who knows a tsunami is coming her way but there is no longer any time to outrun it.

Part Two

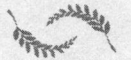

Pre-Op

FOURTEEN

Unheard Stories

When I begin to tell friends about my upcoming surgery, they respond with their own stories. It seems that people have untold stories just waiting to be shared, and the stories come pouring in. But I'm feeling relieved mostly, not sad. Even though this is a safe-ish operation, some of my friends have had complications and share them. I don't necessarily want to hear them. This operation doesn't spell trouble for me. It spells the end of my trouble, or so I hope.

ONE FRIEND CALLS and says, "I don't want to frighten you but . . ." and then tells me horrifying details from her surgery gone wrong.

Another friend phones me. She's been drinking maybe and keeps saying, "I had a hysterectomy and it was no big deal. But I've *had* kids, so I don't even know what kind of road *you're* walking down." She says it so many times that I finally just hold the phone away from my head for a few minutes.

Poor everybody, right?

I get that mourning isn't something you move through, that it's more like something you come back to over and over and over again. It's recursive, and I'm old enough now to suspect that no one ever really gets over anything.

Each person's grief is an ocean wide, forced into a thimble.

sound of my sneakers in the gravel. I'd just walk up their hill into the cool darkness, let my lungs stretch out, be away from the road, burn off my nerves, and try to get a little bit stronger before surgery, if I can. Walking up into their woods seems a way to make peace with things.

HERE'S WHAT I write in the card to the monks. I call them *Brothers* but find out later that I should have referred to them as *Fathers*. Oh well. I tried.

> Dear Brothers,
>
> I am writing to you because I have just learned that I will need surgery in a few weeks. I'm looking for a place to walk now, to try and get stronger before I go into the hospital.
>
> Afterward I will need a place to walk too, to get strong again. I won't be allowed to drive for a while, and our road is too wild for walking (as you no doubt know), with no shoulder and furious New Jersey drivers.
>
> I am hoping you might allow me to walk up your driveway and along the road to your abbey every day or so for a few weeks.

FIFTEEN

Writing to the Monks

When I get the date for surgery, I go to my box of note cards and write to the monks who live nearby. I have never met them, but I've seen the sign on the road for their abbey, and once I saw them: men in black robes and black hats standing by their mailbox. *Greek Orthodox*, I think, not knowing what that means, not even knowing if that is correct.

As I fall asleep the last couple of nights, I find myself fantasizing about walking along the road to the monks' mailbox and then up their long driveway into the woods. There is a big hill there that goes up into the trees, and it looks cool and dark and peaceful. I want to tell the monks that if they let me in, I would be respectful, but that sounds idiotic and like what someone who is disrespectful might say to cover up their disrespectfulness, the way a total player keeps saying, "Trust me." I want to tell the monks that I wouldn't litter or pick their flowers. I wouldn't make any noise other than the

I SIGN IT with my name, our phone number, and *Your neighbor* next to our address. I don't know what they'll think. I don't know if the neighborhood has been kind or unkind to them. And, of course, I've never reached out to them until I wanted something from them, which embarrasses me.

THREE HOURS AFTER I put the card in their mailbox, the phone rings. Craig and I are watching TV. It's dark out. A voice says into my ear, "This is Archbishop J." He hesitates. "I got your letter today and was afraid I'd lose your phone number, so I've called right away."

"Hello," I say, shocked that he called at all, much less so soon, much less that he's an archbishop. Seems overkill.

"You're welcome here," he says. *Pause pause pause.* "And come in for water after your walks, or to rest." I can tell he is uneasy by the way he pauses, and by the way that, as soon as I am ready to say something, he awkwardly interrupts and then pauses again. But he seems happy that someone has asked for something he can provide. He is eager to help and shy about helping at the same time. It's sweet. He reminds me of many men I know who love simply to be useful in the world.

"Be careful of the bears on Thursday mornings," the archbishop says. "That's when the garbage goes out." Of course, I already know that. We live just a few driveways away, but there might as well be a thousand miles between us, we are such complete strangers. "The bears must know, because they come out on Thursday mornings when the garbage goes out. So be careful, and make a lot of noise on Thursdays." *Pause pause pause*. "If you do walk then."

"I'll be careful." I'm smiling.

"And our road is uneven. There are rocks and potholes."

"I'll bring a walking stick a friend has lent me."

"Oh good, that's just the thing."

I don't like asking for help, I never do it, but as I click off my phone, and fill Craig in on the conversation, I start to get a sense that there will be unexpected benefits from this illness. I picture the monks waiting all these years by their mailbox for a card that asks them for a favor, and now that the card has finally arrived, they can be the good neighbors they have been waiting to become. The surgery has forced me to ask for help, also leading me to new friends, to a new place to walk, to new adventures, however circumscribed they might be.

When I get off the phone with the archbishop, I'm left with the sense that the very cells making up the exploded universe want me to be well again, want me to ask for and take the help that is offered.

SIXTEEN

To the Abbey

hemoglobin (hee-muh-gloh-bin, hem-uh): the oxygen-carrying pigment of red blood cells that gives them their red color and serves to convey oxygen to the tissues

—Dictionary.com

The next day, despite thick blood, exhaustion, and the dull ache that twists behind my guts like a slow-moving river, I put on the maxi-est pad I can find, get my walking stick, and walk, for the first time since Craig and I moved here a decade ago, all the way to the abbey, deep in the woods.

I am excited to be somewhere I've never been before, to be doing something new and awkward, quiet and solitary. Perhaps I'll meet the monks in their long black robes. How many live here?

The thought of making new friends even now, at age fifty-two, is nourishing to me. Even sick and unmoored, waiting for surgery, even tired and breathless, there are new friends down the road, in the woods. It's stunning.

When I come to the monks' mailbox, I turn into the shade of their driveway, which is so long (and rutted) that I can't see the end of it from the road. The first part is a steep uphill climb, steep for me, anyway, with my low hemoglobin levels that manifest mostly in me being easily fatigued.

THE TOP OF the hill sits beneath enormous maple trees, making cool green shade where three driveways branch off in different directions. On the right-most driveway is a handwritten sign that reads Abbey (with an arrow), so I walk along the hilly dirt road. I can see how high I've climbed by looking down at the road far below, visible between the trees. There are bittersweet vines slowly swallowing entire trees. There are enormous rocks coming up out of the leaf litter, like whales breaching.

There's a trailer parked at the end of the driveway, and a little construction site with what looks like the white of freshly poured concrete, and beyond that a house with rust-brown shutters, which may be the abbey itself. I pass by an old station wagon that has Wendy's cups in the cup holders. The monks are not ghosts. They are real people who get Cokes at Wendy's. They have given me structure for my days, a place to breathe in the just-turning leaves, a place from which I can head back toward home. It is a place where the silent eyes of restless bears and praying monks can bear witness to the slow-motion shipwreck I'm in the midst of.

Regardless of the fact that this is not a dangerous surgery, I think about death even more than I usually do. He's just sort of with me at the moment, and I don't mind.

It's probably melodrama to think about death, or maybe it's just wanting to acknowledge and minimize my own fears right now, but I figure that if I had to die here, in the leaves under the trees, well, it's as holy a place as any, a witnessed place. Anywhere along this walk in the woods would be a fine place to die, if it came to that. The squirrels and blue jays, the poison ivy, the drying-up stream would together be enough friendship to make it a fine place for a final exhalation up into the sky.

I am afraid of plenty, afraid of discomfort, of pain, of what I worry might be the disorientation of grave illness. I'm afraid of being a burden, afraid of being taken care of by strangers, but Death? No, I'm not afraid of that. I prefer to allow Death in than to pretend he isn't standing just over there. He's not the worst companion I've had. He isn't menacing. He doesn't give unsolicited advice (the thing that annoys me the most). He isn't even slightly judgmental. No. He just feels like the coming winter when the mallards leave so that they can return in the spring. He is as much a friend as my long-gone grandmother, as much a friend as the monks or as the specks of stars clustering around the bowl of the moon.

In the driveway by the abbey, there is a man in a black robe and skullcap picking up old bricks and putting them into a dumpster. "Hello," I say, and introduce myself.

"Yes, Archbishop J told me about you. We will pray for you."

This man's shy, open-armed manner makes me smile, makes me think, *Look at what asking has brought me.*

SEVENTEEN

Calendars

I take out Grandma Hastings' little Norcross calendar, the one I've looked at now and then over the years. On one corner she's written a small shopping list: *Alka Seltzer, face soap, comb*. Did her stomach hurt? Is that why she needed Alka Seltzer?

Every day I write in my own calendar how much I am bleeding. *lite* or *heavy*. Some days I write *very lite* to indicate that *something* is happening. It is as close to *not bleeding* as I get lately.

Everything's getting muddled together—Monday becomes Tuesday in my mind. When you're sick, it's hard to remember being well. When you're well, you assume you'll always be well. Sick and well are thus walled off from one another. I find it hard to peek up and look beyond this one moment.

I still have a vague hope for days in my calendar that will read *no bleeding*, which doesn't happen anymore. I flip back a few pages to check. Right. Hasn't happened for a long time.

I bleed all the time, every day now.

FIRST LIFT IN ENERGY, Grandma Hastings wrote on the back of February 1969.

EIGHTEEN

Keeping Track of Days

I make a note in my calendar when I walk to the abbey. I walk down my road to their driveway, then up the steep one hundred or so steps, then along the gravel road of their long final driveway, in the gray of these September mornings.

In my calendar, Monday reads, *very very lite*, and just beneath that I've scribbled, *abbey—father enoch*, because I was bleeding just a little when I met Father Enoch by the bell tower they are building.

Devout little atheist that I am, I cannot help being moved when he says, "We are praying for you." He has memorized the date of my surgery. He will pray. Love is love, and I'll drink it from a stream or from an old paper cup, I don't care which. In fact, I'd prefer cups that I can't break, that I don't need to wash. Everything's too much for me lately, and I no longer see why I would fight off love.

NINETEEN

Damming Up Streams

While the idea of visiting the monks comforts me, I remain an introvert who prefers the quiet life of my little circle of family, garden, cats, the bugs in the garden, the iris corms that I dig up and separate each fall. The only person I like to hug is Craig, and formal clothes give me hives. Not just now. As far back as I can remember. Dressing up has never been my thing.

People who are not me are willing to talk with strangers about a lot of intimate stuff. Total strangers will tell me how many kids I ought to have had or how much I should weigh or why my name (West) irritates them. But not many people talk about *this* stuff, the miscarriages and hysterectomies, the failures, the ways we feel we've fallen short, the messes we've made.

So, despite my initial reticence, I post online that I'm going to have a hysterectomy. Now it's not just a few close friends who know but dozens of acquaintances (and even some strangers) chime in to tell me, to tell the world perhaps for the first time, "I had one too." I get emails and phone calls from people who want to tell me that they are part of the silent, hysterectomied masses. It pushes me back into my chair. I would never have known, and so what I worried was a bit too personal to share, feels like the right thing to have done. I am not alone. They are not alone.

A few days later, cards start to arrive. I save each one in a basket to show Mom. Her family hailed from New Orleans, and she has retained some of that patience that the South can instill in a person. She reads people's letters with care and pleasure, and she handwrites letters back to them, one at a time, on beautiful cards made by artists. So I save my cards in a MacDowell basket. To my own surprise, I read and reread them. I read the cards people send with care. It amazes me how happy they make me. Why am I usually such a curmudgeon? Why am I always in such a hurry? These cards are lovely. I must remember to send people more handwritten letters.

People reach out and ask how they can help, and similar to many times when people have asked me that, I can't think of anything for anyone to do. The truth is that I have pretty much everything I need: a sweet husband, health insurance, just enough money in the bank and from unemployment (thank god) to pay my bills, for right now anyway. My mother is near enough that she can help. No, I can't think of anything I need.

But my mother, still that New Orleans girl at heart, raised me to never turn down a gift. "That's just rude," she says, and I know she's right. "When someone offers you a gift, you take it. You open it in front of them. You make a fuss. You thank them." She doesn't look tough, with her curled-under blond (now white) hair, but she can take you down, I don't care how spry you think you are. Her certainty about how life ought to work is reassuring. I, on the other hand, am not sure of one single thing ever. Certainty must skip a generation.

Because of her admonitions, I invent something for people to do. When someone wants to know what they can do to help, I ask them to trace their hands and cut out the shapes, and send them to me, and they do, by the dozens. I tape them up on the wall over the new daybed that we've set up in the sunroom, where I'll sleep after surgery. What was at first just me giving people something to do becomes important to me, becomes part of my preparation for surgery. I picture getting home from the hospital and convalescing in the daybed while I look up and see all of my friends' hands there. It's comforting already as I tape one after another to the wall, some tiny ones from little kids, some big ones on black paper, some with notes written on them, some from friends, some from people I've never met. It's corny maybe, but I choose to let it in. Cynicism at this moment seems overrated.

Then the boxes start to arrive, twenty, thirty, forty. I didn't realize that I knew this many people. Books arrive from friends (I read every single one eventually), and candles, healing CDs, chocolate, scented pens, hand-knit neck warmers, a teddy bear, even Goldenberg's Peanut Chews. Almost every day a box arrives (or maybe two or three), a little one sometimes, and once or twice a big one with lots of tape holding it together. Even the unopened boxes are nice, just sitting there on the kitchen counter. This is the perfect way for me to socialize . . . via US mail.

People call too, to chat, to tell me about their surgeries, to send their support. I've never let this kind of thing in before, never knew it was there, was never interested in it, shunned it even.

Well, I'm interested now.

WHEN I WAS a kid my sister and I would spend summer afternoons damming up small streams in the Westchester woods near our home. It was a lot of work because the water always found its way around a twig, a clot of grass, a stone. And that's how this feels, like damming up all of this outpouring is pointless. It will find its way to me no matter what I do. So I stop trying to block it. I just let it flow toward me, and it feels good to be a human being, cared for by other human beings.

I can't remember why I would ever have wanted to shut this out in the first place—maybe the corniness of it? Maybe the hive-inspiring attention? I simply can't imagine. I should have invited all of my friends to our wedding instead of being such a nervous wreck.

It occurs to me that there is something about me not needing anything that makes people especially generous. It's the needy people we shy away from, ironically, the people who are always reaching toward us who make us lean away. I sit in my chair with the cats nearby, my husband on his way home from work. He will inevitably make me laugh, as he does every day over and over. He will hold up the corner of the blanket to invite me into our bed. All of this means that, really, I need nothing, and so here it comes pouring toward me like an avalanche.

TWENTY

A Crack in Me the Size of the World

As surgery draws closer, my focus narrows and deepens. I can go out, can go for walks to the abbey, or for short trips to the grocery store, say, but I am bleeding so hard that I'd rather be home. I am using up giant pads every hour of every day at this point, and I'm exhausted, and also aware that I am on the verge of a huge mess. I think in images more and think about how illness affects how we perceive the world, how illness might shape an artist's mind. I write a poem, the first one I've ever written and I am sure it's not good, but I have something I want to express. I'm writing to tell myself how I feel.

There's a crack in me
the size of the world
made of my parents' sighing and leaning into one
    another

and widened by the hummingbird in the trumpet
   vine

Made wider
   by the smell of my husband's neck in the dark
   and of possible futures crackled and blown away

The crack is unfillable
   like a bottomless pitcher under an open hose
   or a mudslide pouring forever into a sinkhole

Everything tumbles into me:
   the hummingbird
   my parents' sighs
   blown-away sorrows
until I am ecstatic over loss and gain

The tears of laughter and the tears of shattered
   everythings
gather and collect and fracture and rise
regardless of whether I believe in them or not
Mattering so very little is pure delight.

TWENTY-ONE

Along the Path

Along the path to the abbey there is sometimes a straw hat hanging from a branch, or maybe there is *always* a hat and I only notice it some mornings. I am not as aware as I wish I were, and days confuse me, each spilling into the next or the prior one. My brain refuses to understand time and logistics lately, seems unable to focus on the quotidian, on the items found on a To Do list. Can low iron levels do that?

But as some things fall away, my awareness of other things, like the natural world, sharpens. I notice the squirrels rustling through the poison ivy, the late summer stream all dried up waiting for a storm to fill it. I am more attuned to this kind of thing than I think I've ever been. The busy larger world has fallen away. It is me and the streams now, me and my breath.

I like the sweetness of the monks in the abbey, dandruff in their beards. I like the way they pray for me, and the way the natural world seems to vibrate around me as my storm comes on.

GRANDMA STOPPED WRITING in her calendar, I assume, because she died. Soon, in a few months maybe, I will not be writing in my calendar about blood or walks for a different reason. I think about what I will be keeping track of—the rusted barbell that sits beneath that pine tree? The snow that is surely on its way? Or maybe I will forget to write in my calendar at all. Monday will not say *heavy bleeding* because once the bleeding stops, there will no longer be anything to keep track of.

TWENTY-TWO

Shade

A hundred-year-old pine fell down at my mother's house a year or two ago. It was a sorrow to all of us. We knew that tree, had grown up next to it. It had been a home to owls and vultures and peregrine falcons who'd perched in its branches way up by our bedroom windows. Its pinecones had been harassed by hungry squirrels who dropped them on our cars like torpedoes.

But the tree was old, its roots weakened by the decades, and the wind and rain of some particular hurricane finally knocked it over. A year or two later, you'd hardly know there had been a tree there, the ground where it fell is so full of riotous greenery.

Skunks waddle through the tangled underbrush at night. Deer raise up on their hind legs to reach the sweet lower branches of new growth. There are cardinals who nest there, and probably moles and worms wriggling underneath.

I LOOK FORWARD to seeing what will sprout after the
doctors snip out my uterus, and cut away its fallopian
tube branches, take away the root of the cervical muscle.
Surely something has been lying in the shade of all this
grief.

IT WAS ONLY after Dad died that I saw how large a
shadow he'd cast. He would have laughed at the way I
flourished when his death made room for me.

I remember beating him at Scrabble when I was in
third grade, and he went around telling anyone who
would listen, "She trounced me!" So, it's not like he
planned on casting a shadow over his kids, it's not like
it was intentional.

But Dad had a lot of personality. He was the tallest
tree in the family and got all the light, and my roots
learned to grow down deep and quiet to get what they
needed.

On my walks now, I think about what lies in the
shade of what the doctors are taking out of me. What
will grow tall when my uterus and the antennae of
my fallopian tubes have been carved away? Nothing?
Everything?

Something unexpected will come, and I will be

looking for it, looking forward to walking the path beside what grows in its place.

I wish I could have both walked beside my father *and* been in the bright sunshine that only his death afforded.

And he would have loved that too, I feel pretty sure.

TWENTY-THREE

Instructions on My Death

I dream about the family tomb in New Orleans, the aboveground one where my mother's family is buried. Dad is buried there now too with Mom's mom, Grandma Hastings, and I'll probably end up there as well, my ashes snug amidst everyone else's bones and dust.

Most everyone is all paired up there. My maternal great-great-grandmother, Mary Bella Brice, is with her second husband, A. G. Brice. Her daughter and son-in-law are there too. (They died young of I don't know what.) But Grandma Hastings was buried spouseless. I went not long ago to visit my grandfather's grave way up near the Canadian border in Constable, New York, where he grew up. I think that the happiest times of his troubled life were up there. He's buried there next to their baby girl who lived, as Grandma used to say, "just long enough for me to make a scrapbook for her." I had found a lock of Grandma's hair in an envelope in an attic box, which I left at this baby's gravesite. Her name was Mary. She also lived long enough to be named.

But way, way back, before she married my grandfather, when Grandma Hastings was Rosina West, a girl of nineteen or so, she was in love with someone else entirely. His name was Horton, and I found his obituary at the Historic New Orleans Collection a few years ago. She was in love with him and he killed himself. The headline of the obituary reads that Horton "Put a Bullet in His Brain." After Grandma died, my mother was visiting New Orleans and asked a friend of Grandma's what had happened with Horton back in 1914. Why did a man of such promise kill himself?

"Oh, darling," said Jeanne Sully Floweree West (no relation) over martinis, "Horton put a gun to his head and blew his brains out. He'd learned he had syphilis, Annie. He didn't want to shame your poor mother."

Of course, none of *that* was in Horton's obituary.

But I imagine that it was because of her great love for Horton that Grandma was buried alone in the family tomb in New Orleans. The man she would go on to marry, my grandfather, was a disappointment, I think. He died of cirrhosis of the liver in his fifties after "pissing away the family fortune," as my mother puts it. He chose to be buried near the Saint Lawrence River, where he fished for muskellunge as a boy, far away from his wife in New Orleans, but next to the little baby girl who lived only a week or so. The way everyone is scattered makes me feel like a bell without a clapper.

MOST PEOPLE DON'T talk easily about death, but in my family, we talk about death the same way other families talk about groceries or the weather.

I don't want Craig to worry, so I tell him, "If I die while they are operating on me, that's a good thing." After watching my father's slow death, his falling to pieces, I figure that if I happen to die while anesthetized on an operating table, hell! That seems like the most pain-free death a person could wish for. No suffering. No suffering is the brass ring of dying, right?

Craig ignores my talk of death. It's not like I want to die. There are wrinkly rhubarb leaves to watch unfurl in early spring. Given my way, I'd live forever if I could watch those leaves push up from the just-thawed dirt every spring. And I have books to write. I have reasons to live.

IT HELPS TO talk about the worst-case scenario, though, and I wonder why families don't discuss it. I've seen friends tell their dying mothers:, "No, no, you'll be fine, don't talk like that." That seems a cruel thing to say to someone who wants to tell you that they're afraid. I guess maybe it feels better sometimes to pretend that Death isn't coming for the people we love. I get that. Sort of.

If I am to die during this surgery—and that is very unlikely—I'd like someone to go into the woods to let the leaves and the squirrels and the pebbles know not to expect me. That is the kind of thing I think about as I walk in the woods a week before surgery, how sad it would be to never stand in the forest again, to never again see September wrench into October. The earth. I want more time with the earth.

Yes, I'm an atheist, but I kind of like the idea of ending up in Metairie Cemetery in New Orleans with all of those gone family members. I like to imagine that one day, when I get to the family tomb, we can set up a card table and have some drinks. I'll finally get to meet my great-great-grandmother Mary Bella Brice, whose paintings hung on the walls of my childhood home. Her husband, the stern-looking Judge A. G. Brice, with the long white pointy beard, would be there too, along with Dad and Grandma Hastings. You have to admit, it sounds a little bit like fun, doesn't it? But wouldn't it be nice if I could meet Horton too, who's buried somewhere else in New Orleans, and Grandma's little baby girl, and even my alcoholic grandfather, the one who pissed away the family fortune? I'd like even him. He was a fellow author, writing a weekly column for the *Christian Science Monitor* for decades. He wore spats, for god's sake, and smoked cork-tipped cigarettes. I'd like to have a drink with him too, but he was buried up in Constable with Grandma's little week-old baby girl.

TWENTY-FOUR

Grief-y Happiness

A few years after our last miscarriage, Craig and I were lying on our bed one day, on top of the covers with our clothes on, holding hands, staring at the ceiling. We'd been grieving hard for some time over our ability to get pregnant and our inability to carry a pregnancy to term. We had decided, once and for all, that it was time to stop trying to have kids. There were many reasons, not the least of which was my physical exhaustion from three failed pregnancies. I didn't think I could do it again, but we felt an enduring pall over it that pervaded everything, and which was unspoken except between the two of us. We thought about it all the time but found no mechanism to share what we were going through outside of our marriage.

We lay there looking at the ceiling, silent, our warm palms together. Then Craig propped himself up on an elbow and said, "Hey, what if we just tried to be happy anyway? I mean, we can't make the sadness go away, but maybe we can be happy too, at the same time?"

It turns out he was right, as he so often is. We started saying yes to things, to barbecues and walks, to baby showers even, and it turns out you can be filled to overflowing with grief and still be happy.

IT WAS AFTER Craig suggested that we might be happy despite everything that I made a secret decision. I'd never felt a hunger for children until I became pregnant, but being pregnant over and over again had awoken a fierce desire in me to create something lasting.

One morning, when Craig had just gotten out of the shower, I said to him:, "I have something to tell you, but don't tell anyone else, OK?"

"OK," he said, wrapping a towel around his waist, and grabbing his toaster waffle from the toaster oven.

"I'd like to see if I can really be a writer."

THAT WAS EIGHT or nine years ago, and now that it's time for my uterus to be removed, I am not feeling griefed up hardly at all about my childlessness. Scared of the surgery? Yes, I'm feeling scared, but I am not grieving over this, or not at the moment I'm not. Or not wildly. Or not consciously.

I feel a little bit defensive about it, like I should be upset or something, but today I am not sorrowful about my uterus being gone. In fact, the idea of never bleeding again sounds like pure heaven, in a low-hemoglobin kind of way. The idea of not bleeding anymore seems really sweet, really worth anything, worth everything in fact. And it seems like my best bid for happiness.

I do not think, *Boo-hoo. Without a uterus, I am no longer a woman.* Nope. I project out to a week after surgery and think, *There will be a time, quite soon, when you won't be bleeding anymore.*

TWENTY-FIVE

Questions for My Doctor

The doctor is calling tomorrow to answer any pre-op questions I might have. In trying to behave like a well-informed and thoughtful patient, I sit down to make a list of questions about anesthesia and recovery time. But each time I write something serious—Should I stop taking my vitamins? for instance—I write something that makes me laugh.

Finally I give up, and this is what I write on my yellow legal pad instead.

THINGS TO DISCUSS WITH MY DOCTOR BEFORE THE HYSTERECTOMY

1. How long until I can:
   • Drive
   • Shower
   • Have sex
   • Drink gin

- Lie in the hammock
- Be annoyed at my neighbor for wearing a Nazi-style motorcycle helmet
- Be annoyed at everyone in the world like they deserve

2. Is diving down into the netherworld between my legs, through the speculum and into my widened cervix, like time travel at all? Is it like Jules Verne's *Journey to the Center of the Earth*? Or *10,000 Leagues Under the Sea*, maybe?
   - Is there a moment when you're horrified by the sheer biology of an inert, naked, middle-aged woman in that outrageous position?
   - Does it look anything like the star-nosed mole that scared the living crap out of me in my garden last summer, all twitchy, whiskery and blind?
   - Have I now ruined star-nosed moles for you?

3. Truth is I've never been fond of vaginas. I picture mine looking like Winston Churchill's vagina, if he had been a woman, or maybe Mrs. Doubtfire's vagina. I apologize ahead of time if mine looks like Mrs. Doubtfire's British, middle-aged man-vagina.
   - Also, why do you suppose the two examples I've

given of vaginas above are of men's vaginas?

- Also, also "vagina" is a terrible word.
- Also, also, ALSO please don't show these questions to anyone.

4. Do you have a periscope?
   - Do you wish you had a periscope?
   - Do you sometimes fantasize about wearing a submarine captain's uniform while you operate?
   - Do you eat a big can of spinach before operating, the way Popeye would?
   - Why do I equate this surgery with naval exercises?

5. What are the things that can go wrong?
   - What are the things that can go horribly wrong?
   - Do you sometimes wish you had just gone to pharmacy school?

6. During the operation could we listen to Bach's "Goldberg Variations"?
   - And right before you put me under, will you hold my hand and look into my face and smile?
   - Just stand there until I close my eyes, if you would, so that my last image might be of a competent human being.

- Not to be bossy, but smile with your eyes because I won't be able to see your mouth behind the surgical mask.
- And don't play Vivaldi. That fucker makes my heart race.

LATER, I WANT to show this list to my doctor, but by the time I think of it, I am too sick and he is too busy. When it's all over (and he retires soon after I recover), I realize that he never saw it and I no longer know how to reach him. Oh well. I guess it wasn't meant for him.

TWENTY-SIX

Checking Under the Hood

Today I take my car in to get an oil change. It's the kind of task I can still do because it shouldn't take me far from home, and I'm trying to get everything on earth taken care of before surgery. So I take my car to a place three miles from home to Josh, a guy I know and trust, for an oil change (a thousand miles early), and they can't open the hood. It's been a problem for a while, but now the problem has come home to roost, and I need to face it. Time has run out.

Next, I take the car to a body shop ten miles away, and the guy with an oil smudge over one eyebrow can't open it either. I have this stuffed-down, frantic feeling that I am going to get this motherfucking hood open and the oil changed on this car no matter what it takes. I'm not going to leave this mess for after surgery, or for someone else to deal with. So I take it to the dreaded VW dealership where everything costs a fortune, and for $302 (plus tax), they open the stupid hood.

TWENTY-SEVEN

Under the Hood

cervix (SER-vix): The lower, narrow end of the uterus
that forms a canal between the uterus and vagina.

—Cancer.gov

My doctor called today, after I got home from the hood odyssey, to answer my actual, real pre-op, one-week-before-surgery questions.

I'd been looking at material online about exactly how these vaginal hysterectomies are done, and it looked to me as though they'd cut right through the cervix to get to the uterus, but I wasn't sure. I'd been thinking that a vaginal hysterectomy had such a quick recovery specifically because it did not require cutting through any muscle fiber, but I'm pretty sure the cervix is a muscle, so I ask him, "Will you cut through my cervix?"

"I'm *removing* your cervix." He says it like it's obvious, and it is in the definition I'd found, so I guess I just didn't take in the meaning before this conversation. (I learn later that removing the cervix *is* pretty routine, but I don't know that at the time, and when I do realize it, I feel like someone should clarify that for us lay people. Why do people assume we know things that we couldn't possibly just know?)

Jesus. I hadn't expected that they were going to remove my cervix. Like a door slammed, I flinch.

I don't think I will miss my uterus. It's problematic, diseased. I've never seen it. But my cervix—my cervix I know with my fingertips from situating my diaphragm there back in the eighties. And now it will be gone . . . a piece of me that I can visualize will be gone. This feels different, worse than the actual hysterectomy, which carried almost zero emotional baggage.

The silky, slippery nose of my cervix, who never did anything to anyone, cannot apparently be saved, and for some idiotic reason I'm sitting here, alone in the living room by my bowl of popcorn feeling horrible, as though I have not been a good steward for my body, as though I can't protect this innocent almost-creature from the onslaught.

The day is a bust. I won't be able to sleep now, and even worse, although they got the hood open on my car,

I never even got the oil change because sometimes even the smallest things are so much harder than you expect them to be.

AFTER A WHILE, I look up *cervix* on WebMD and learn that "The part of the cervix that can be seen from inside the vagina during a gynecologic examination is known as the ectocervix. An opening in the center of the ectocervix, known as the external os, opens to allow passage between the uterus and vagina." The language of it is cool and soothing. "*External os*," I say out loud.

Turns out that the "overlapping border between the endocervix and ectocervix is called the transformation zone." Neat.

I've never seen or touched my uterus or fallopian tubes, and so their imminent removal is vague, intangible, theoretical. But the fact that my cervix, something that I know, will be cut away, changes everything. No longer knowing my own internal geography has me disoriented.

TWENTY-EIGHT

Unstoppable Things

Tonight in bed, I am full-on frightened for the first time, so I picture myself like a little lamb being hugged very close, my eyes shut tight, my face rubbed and rubbed by loving fingers.

But then . . . my cervix, and I'm awake again. Funny the things that bother me and the things that don't. Death is fine but don't take my cervix. What a weirdo.

I close my eyes again, and this time I picture myself as a tiny grain of sand on the beach beneath an enormous black sky dotted with stars. My eyes close and my husband snores and I almost drift off.

But then . . . my cervix, and I'm awake again.

I reach for my glasses to sneak out and write, but instead of finding my glasses in the dark, I knock over the moisturizer, which clatters loudly to the floor, and ask myself the question I ask almost every night: Why don't I ever put my glasses in the same spot?

Craig wakes up at the noise and squints at the clock. "Ah, twelve thirty-four is a good time to get up—one-two-three-four."

He loves numbers, and nothing I do is wrong to him. But I hate to wake him. "Shhhh," I say. "You're dreaming." I can feel him smile in the dark as I creak out of bed.

The moon is shining so bright that it casts shadows in the room. The gossamer curtain over the bedroom window makes the breeze visible. It blows in at me softly, like we are all ghosts.

I SIT DOWNSTAIRS and write. It is now 1:11, *one-one-one*, a good time to be up. I hear my husband snore, curled in our bed upstairs like a cashew. I feel my father in the sky, hanging inside the moon and watching. Years ago I was in the recovery room with Dad after he had open-heart surgery. As he woke up, he clutched my hand. "I woke up in the middle of the operation," he croaked, still terrified, close to tears. "The tube was down my throat, and I couldn't tell them, but I was awake. I was awake." If he *is* in the moon, maybe he is pondering what I will make of my life after the surgery.

Or maybe he is wondering what I'll make of my life

period. I wonder that myself, often. I haven't made much of it yet, no kids, a stalled career.

I know one thing for sure—I do not want them to take my cervix, and frantically wish that I could keep it. But it may as well already be gone.

And I do not want to be intubated either, but I can already feel the tube lodged in my constricting throat. Things, unstoppable things, have been set in motion.

If only I would put my glasses in the same place every night, maybe things would be simpler. I could find them then, in the dark, without disturbing my peaceful husband.

TWENTY-NINE

Growing Up

Nothing is what I thought it would be when I was young.

I was a worrier from the get-go, but back when I was a kid it never occurred to me that my hair would be anything but glossy, that I'd ever be anything but promise and forward momentum.

No one explains anything about growing up or growing old to you, or maybe they do and we just don't listen. It wouldn't matter if they did. Who could believe any of it, and who could go on knowing what lay ahead?

THIRTY

Curl of Smoke

By five years old, I was already an insomniac. I couldn't read, so I didn't yet have books as late-night companions, and the quieting down of the house around me made me feel frightened, like I was by myself in the vast universe of darkness.

After Grandma Hastings moved in, when I couldn't sleep, I would take a journey in the dead of night, creeping down the long hallway past my brother's room, my sister's room, the hallway that led to Mom and Dad's room, down the thirteen stairs (holding the banister with my fingertips for balance), past the living room, and finally to Grandma Hastings' door, where she'd tacked that picture of a dove holding an olive branch in its beak.

At night Grandma looked different, ethereal. Her gray hair, which was up in a tight, neat bun during the day, would be unwound and flowed like gossamer down below her waist. In the dark she had the silhouette of a girl . . . or of a ghost. I would say quietly from the doorway, "Grandma? I can't sleep," and she would say, "Come get into bed." I would climb under the covers, and then she'd tell me a story, one with no action, to calm me. It was usually about a cottage in Ireland with a thatched roof, a cottage that had a tidy dirt floor that was swept clean every morning. If you walked away from the cottage and looked back at it, she said, you could see a curl of smoke coming from the chimney. Grandma rested her hand on my back as she told me about the curl of smoke, about the swept-dirt floor, about the thatched roof where flowers might grow. I didn't know that she was sick, that she was wearing a back brace. What do children know but their own little worries?

And when she had calmed me, and I was no longer despairing, she would send me back to my own bed, where I would think about the thatched-roof cottage with its swept-dirt floor until I fell asleep.

Once Dad got sick, he and Mom moved downstairs to Grandma Hastings' old room, and my mother never moved out. She sleeps in that room now, older than her mother ever lived to be. My mother lives in Grandma Hastings' old room, the room that once had the picture of the dove thumb-tacked to its door.

THIRTY-ONE

The Path to the Abbey

I've been to the abbey every day since the arch-bishop called. The monks are building a bell tower up there out of bricks, and sometimes I see Father Enoch trying to tidy up and get all the construction debris into the dumpster. He has a red beard, and I question how old he is. He could be twenty. He could be thirty-five.

It has been three days since I've seen the hat hanging on the branch. I've been really paying attention, so I guess it's gone, but I ask myself if I am overlooking it each time or is it really no longer hanging on the branch?

There is a rusted exhaust pipe in the woods that is pretty, the brown rust making it look like a bent branch.

There is a rock by the side of the road that has other little rocks on it, and I wonder if someone is putting little rocks on the bigger rock, or did the spinning tire of a car cough up the gravel?

I want to be in conversation with what is around me, so I decide I will put another rock on top of that other rock every time I walk past it. But then I think that it is vanity to need to leave a mark on things. Who cares if I walk this way, or if I don't?

Still, maybe tomorrow I will add a rock to the pile just to see if a squirrel will notice, or if it might make the hat return to the branch, or maybe just to see if it will help me see the hat on the branch that has been there all the time. There is no reason to stop being playful.

THIRTY-TWO

Where Are the Grown-Ups?

mantis ('man(t)əs) (also *praying mantis*): A slender predatory insect related to the cockroach. It waits motionless for prey with its large spiky forelegs folded like hands in prayer.

—Lexico.com

When Craig and I got married and bought our house, it was the first one for either of us. The closing was harrowing, as many closings are. We realized we had to come up with a thousand unexpected bucks for the oil in the tank, for instance. Jesus. After signing checks and contracts, we went for a drink down the road at the Town Tavern (closed now) and slumped over the bar, spent. Afterwards, when we walked into the empty house that night, our house now, we turned to each other and said, "When the hell are the grown-ups coming home?" We were both in our forties.

A COUPLE OF days before the surgery, my eighty-four-year-old mom comes out from her home in Westchester, an hour away, to stay with us. It's a warm September, and we decide that she and I will live together in the sunroom when I return from the hospital. We've set up the daybed for me, and the futon-couch for her. She says it's ideal. We will be steps from the kitchen, the coffee machine, the bathroom . . . steps from each other as I convalesce.

My mother loves this room even though it's a bit ramshackle. It's a run-down part of our old farmhouse and is enclosed on three sides with floor-to-ceiling windows so that we can watch wildlife while we sit with our coffee in the morning, with our gin in the evening. We can hear the chickens next door, and sometimes around cocktail time, someone is playing scales on a trumpet. He sounds close, but he could be miles away. I picture the trumpet player as a man, but it could be my long-haired neighbor, the one who talks kindly to her chickens. Trumpet music coming from the woods at cocktail time every night is how life should be. The more oddball the better as far as I'm concerned.

After moving to this house a decade ago, I called my mother when I spotted the first groundhog poking up by the pond. He was so fat I thought maybe he was a beaver. I called her again that first year when I realized that the little blades of green emerging from under the maple tree were lilies of the valley, just like in her yard. It was moving to think that I might be like her in some small way, that my life might echo hers, no matter how faintly. I didn't understand then that she had a particular capacity for happiness that I hadn't inherited. That isn't something you can acquire. You either have it or you don't.

My mother has begun to lose her hearing, and I remember the weight in my chest when I learned that she could no longer hear the spring peepers. The impossible had happened; she had grown old.

This visit of hers is unlike prior visits. She has a bigger bag with more clothes this time. She's brought *books* (plural) to read, and the entire five pounds of her Sunday *New York Times*. We don't know how long she's staying, how long I will need her. "I can stay forever," she says. "Except for my dentist appointment on the fourth." She is rigid like that. No matter how tired she might be, even when Dad was dying, she always made her bed.

There is no excuse in her world for an unmade bed, for a missed appointment, for an unanswered letter.

The sunroom is set up for the expected two weeks or so of my convalescence. But if the doctor has to go in abdominally for some reason, recovery will be weeks longer, so I make sure our shared space is comfy. In addition to the cut-out paper hands from my friends, I've cut zinnias from the garden and filled every single vase I have with them. They line the rickety table at the end of the room. And next to them are the jade plant and the Christmas cactus that was grown from a cutting of Grandma Hastings' cactus.

"Oh my," Mom says, putting her bag down. "Oh," she's leaning over the jade plant. "Look at this!" I lean in and stare, not seeing anything at first, but then, focusing in, I can see she's pointing at a praying mantis.

"Yes," I say, "he's been here a week or two. I named him Claude. Must've brought him in with the zinnias. Bizarre, right?" He is huge and green, fat almost, a full seven inches long. He is alien, weird, still as a coffin, his giant eyes atop his neck-stalk make him look like a 1950s sci-fi movie monster. And yet, I had found him in the sunroom, where the inside of our home and the outside of my garden and our woods converge. I love insects, particularly ants and bees, have an entire shelf of books about insects, but while I admire bugs, I prefer to admire them outside. Ants, for instance, do not fascinate me when they march back and forth to the cat dish, say. But this room is an in-between space, and Claude is welcome here.

"Oh my," my mother says again, clearly fascinated. This love of biology comes from Grandma Hastings, our biologist-debutante from New Orleans. Every time we enter or exit the room, we locate Claude, which takes a minute because of his greenness, and his stillness. And there is that first moment, when we do find him, that is horrifying. To finally have my eyes focus on him in the jade plant, or to find him hanging upside down from the stained-glass window is bloodcurdling, frankly. He is hideous and breathtaking. It is best, probably, not to look too closely at a praying mantis. There is little, if anything, of comfort about them visually, and yet he is our companion and is part of the nest we are building, my mother and I.

With only a few days to go until surgery, my mind continues to change. I seem unable to sustain a thought, or to write anything of length or depth. My mind is active but flitting. It keeps settling back on the praying mantis. I think of Claude as French. The idea of him gives me something of little consequence or duration to think about as I fall asleep. He is gruesome, but I can reduce him, can contain him with humor.

One evening Mom and I are sitting in the darkening sunroom. She gets up to find Claude. Cocktail time is over and the string of solar fairy-lights has come on.

The sky has gone from gray to navy to almost black. We've lit a candle. "He's hanging upside down," she tells me, "perfectly still." I've watched him. He can stand so motionless that he begins to look like the twig he is stuck to.

We're speaking in those quiet voices that are a mixture of gin and dusk. "If he lands in my hair," I whisper, "I'll slap him to death before I even know what I'm doing."

"Of course," she says softly. "Me too."

As I drift off, I think the following to amuse myself:

While a praying mantis is symbolic of patience and stillness, I'm afraid that Claude is not the stillest mantis in the bunch. This may come from too much strong black coffee. Or it could be that his little hands shake from cheap gin and all those late nights as maître d' at Chez Josephine. There are whispers about alcoholism and a case of untreated syphilis from WW II, but we don't listen to rumors any more than we believe in Santa Claus or the Kardashians.

He sometimes breaks into heartrending versions of Edith Piaf songs when the moon is full and the gin bottle is empty. He's not perfect. He most certainly is not. He smokes filter-less Gauloises and snores to shake the rafters. He hates kids and repeats stories from the war. Everyone knows that he's not old enough to have sipped from the trough of forbidden love at Normandy. A mantid lives only one year, but a good story is a good story, and one mustn't allow facts to get in the way.

I'm AWAKE WHEN Mom turns on the outside light in the hope of seeing the feral cat she does not see. She turns off the light. I say, "Good night."

"What?" she asks, turned in my direction.

More loudly now I say, "Good night," and she pauses in a way that lets me know she hasn't heard. I sit up and shout "GOOD NIGHT" at her, which makes us both laugh.

"OK," she says. "Good night." I can hear that she is smiling.

THIRTY-THREE

Hoping

Surgery's in the morning, and I have a wave of thoughts coursing through my brain. I'm hoping to sleep soundly, hoping I don't take a bite of food accidentally after midnight. I lie in the dark, my hands on my chest, my eyes wide-open.

I hope the billion orderlies, phlebotomists, and nurses, the secretaries, janitors, and surgeons, hope everyone I'll come in contact with in the morning doesn't make me cry about anything . . . I hope the monks in the abbey down the road have the right date for this surgery and know when to pray. It's not the prayer that matters to me exactly but their kindness.

I lie in the dark hoping I don't forget too soon what it's been like to be sick . . . I would like to forget (on the other hand) what it's like to bleed for months on end, afraid to go out, exhausted all the time, but I don't want to forget entirely . . . Being ill has made me meet the world with a more patient heart.

I hope that tomorrow morning I crave coffee like I always do, even though I can't have any . . . I want everyone to be nice to Craig . . . I hope that whatever they end up taking out of me makes me healthy . . . I hope I don't say something totally idiotic while I'm coming out of anesthesia . . . Or if I do say something idiotic, that it's at least hilarious . . . I can't wait to see Craig after surgery, and my mom . . . My mom—so happy Mom will be there to help me through this. Me and Mom reading together like when I was a kid so long ago; us whispering to one another in the sunroom with the zinnia-filled vases; the miracle of my body healing around what will be, after tomorrow, an empty pocket.

THIRTY-FOUR

Claude

On the evening before surgery I lie in bed thinking about Claude again. I am getting texts and emails and phone calls from friends and strangers. Everyone is asking how I am and wishing me luck with my surgery, but that is all way too much for me to cope with. I don't know how I am. I'm simultaneously fine, harebrained, and scared, and I don't feel like talking about it or anything else. The people close to me, my deaf mother, my laconic husband, my close friends—they know how I'm feeling as much as anyone can. I trust that no one will mind if I ignore them tonight. I appreciate the invitations, the care. My mind settles on the neutral territory of Claude. I picture him in a tiny beret, nostalgic about his time on the WW II battlefields. He's drunk . . . again, his beret askew. The ash on his Gauloise is precariously long.

Mom is down in the sunroom, one of the cats with her. I assume my mother is asleep on the daybed that

I will be sleeping on tomorrow night. For now, I lie in bed upstairs waiting for Craig, but I don't feel like I am anywhere in particular. When I am not careful, I think about intubation and scalpels, so I drag my mind back to Claude as Craig comes upstairs and brushes his teeth. I imagine Claude misquoting something from *Casablanca*, which strikes me as the funniest thing I've ever heard.

When Craig finally gets into bed, I push my back up against him and sink into the cocoon of his warm arms. He is keeping me safe for now. My eyes blink open, and I look at the fat moon outside my bedroom window. Mom is downstairs, I remind myself, and I feel the ancestors with me too, all of the folks in the family tomb in New Orleans, my father's parents (buried I don't know where). I am their culmination, all of them, and being so confers on me a responsibility to survive the surgery, and to be happy besides. The stories of theirs that survive are housed in me, after all, and so I close my eyes and feel how even the sky is wrapping its arms around me. I think of Grandma Hastings, and her mother, and her mother, on and on and on, and I drift off hugged by Craig and by the nighttime.

THIRTY-FIVE

To Do

I stand in the kitchen, my stomach empty, my body scrubbed clean with antibacterial soap as per instructions. There are pens, books, a comb for the cats in the sunroom. I put my hands on my hips. I've bought kitty litter, vitamins, boxes of tissues, special pricey cold-pressed juices from the health food store (like I'm Jacki O or something), and maxi pads.

Shoot. I should have thrown out the broken picture frame, the one with the jagged glass. I should have wrapped it in newspaper so no one gets cut. I should have written a card to my goddaughter, the one I hardly know, to make sure she understands that she is OK, that it's her father who's messed up.

I've left some things for too long. I won't get to that letter, and I know I won't, even as I remind myself to write it. Some of the things left till the last second are left because they cannot be done anyway.

Then the three of us are in the car on the way to the hospital. "Remember," I tell Craig, "that even if something goes wrong, I do not want to be put on a ventilator." I turn around and shout it at Mom so that she knows too. "I'll take pain meds, though." I wish I could tell Craig right then how much I love our life, even though we're not rich, even though we never had kids, but that would sound like saying goodbye. Plus Mom's in the car, and this is too personal to say in front of her.

"Oh," I say, "do NOT let the funeral home embalm me before cremation. It's a billing scam, plus it's bad for the environment. Put me in a cardboard box, slide me into the oven, push the button, and shove my *cremains* into the family tomb in Metairie with everyone else." I can see in the rearview mirror that Mom hasn't heard. I shout, "I don't want to be embalmed before cremation." She smiles and nods. "Me neither."

I want to remind Craig that Mom simply cannot hear him, that he *has* to enunciate and speak slowly, but of course, now's not the time. I also want to tell him to spend my savings if I die, but saying that seems ridiculous, even though it's what I'm thinking. I am not going to die in this surgery. This surgery is routine, totally routine. They do like half a million of them a year in the US alone. I lean my face against the cold car window. I should have given Craig the passwords for all my accounts, and shown him where my life insurance policy is, oh, and given him the key to our safety deposit box. Too late. Too late. It's too late now for anything, for everything.

If I do live through this, I plan to be selfish. I plan to keep busy writing, and walking in the woods, and drinking gin while listening to that crazy trumpet player next door. When I live through this I hope I'll stop worrying about how much I weigh, and stop worrying about money. Who cares about money? It is the most ridiculous thing to worry about, but I only know this because surgery is so imminent. I will forget again. All I want on the other side of surgery is no more blood, an empty calendar, and a pillow that smells like my husband's neck.

I should have told Craig that I reorganized the pot tops. Dammit. I want credit for that, and now he's going to think Mom did it. Oh well.

THIRTY-SIX

An Untied Balloon

I was led to believe that my womb was sort of the center of me. Jesus, isn't every bit of mascara just a biological imperative meant to help propagate the species? I can see that now. I am more than my procreative capacity. I don't reside in any one place. Even if you cut off my toes, my ankles, my knees, even if you unscrew my casing and pluck out my mechanism, I will still be me, right?

Even when my days are done, my eyes closed and I'm a little packet of ashes in the Louisiana tomb, I will be me, inside the marble, under the Spanish moss. Me. Me. Me. No scalpel can nick that.

Part Three

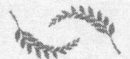

At the Hospital for Surgery

THIRTY-SEVEN

Chilly Rooms

I gave myself a pedicure for surgery, although one without nail polish because I'd heard that it could throw off the oxygen saturation meter that doctors use. If my nailbed turns blue, I want them to be able to see that. I do the pedicure because I want the doctors to think of me as someone who is well tended. I don't know if this makes me slightly pathetic or if it makes me smart. Do doctors notice these things? Can a well-filed toenail make a doctor see me as a human being, even when I'm inert on an operating table? Who knows, but it's like throwing a penny in a fountain. Why not hedge your bets?

I'm also wearing a cute dress because I want every single person I come into contact with in the hospital to see and remember me. I want very much to get better and am aware that I control almost nothing now, so what I can control, I will. I've never taken particularly good care of myself, but the importance of caring for my body has come into sharp focus this morning.

When I am reading stacks of student papers, I can sometimes forget that a human being resides behind the drafts, and I need to wake myself up to the humanity in the lifeless pieces of paper. I want the nurses and doctors and anesthesiologists and physician's assistants and receptionists, the food service personnel, janitors, and secretaries to all be woken up to the humanness beating inside my body. I matter, I want to tell them. I matter.

Mom, Craig, and I have set ourselves up in a little presurgical waiting room. I am looking at the TV without seeing it when Mom and Craig decide to go off and get a bagel and some coffee. The minute they're gone, someone in pale yellow scrubs carrying a clipboard comes to take me away. I don't know how to alert Mom and Craig, so I hesitate and then just follow this stranger. Someone puts a bracelet on me for identification, and I'm told to strip down, put on a gown facing one way or the other, put my things in the hospital locker, and hop up on the gurney.

I am not allowed to wear my underwear, but of course I'm bleeding quite a bit, and so I'm uncomfortable and embarrassed. I ask for a pad to be put under me so that I don't ruin their stuff, and finally someone brings one. The room is chilly. They put an IV in my arm and a shower cap over my hair. A nurse asks me something about my mood, I don't remember the question exactly, but I answer, "I want to live," if that's what she's getting at. The nearness of death is good for that, for making us certain that being alive is where we want to be.

Mom and Craig find me. They come into my little curtained-off, pale yellow "room," and I am relieved. So are they. Craig holds my hand. His feels warm and dry and I can tell by the way he moves his fingers around that he is not relaxed. "We turned around and you were gone," they say.

"I know," I say. I'm grateful to have them with me for this second, knowing that soon we will be pulled in different directions again.

There is an IV dripping saline into me, and I keep thinking that someone should be putting something in the IV to calm me, like the IV equivalent of Xanax. They did that for me before my colonoscopy, so why not now? Even months after the surgery is over, I'm pretty sure I'm right, that someone skipped a step that could have given me a millimeter of extra comfort.

THIRTY-EIGHT

Code Blue

When Dad was dying I asked him, "Do you have any regrets?"

"I wish I had learned to play the piano better," he said, "and I should have found a way for Grandma Hastings to die at home." Although Grandma Hastings was my mother's mother, she and my father came to love one another dearly over the years.

When Grandma went to the hospital for the last time early in 1970, my mother watched as they called a Code Blue on her. A woman in scrubs climbed up onto the bed, straddled Grandma's frail eighty-two-year-old body, and revived her, but at what cost? Grandma was unwell. She had an agonizingly bad back, so bad it required a brace. She was bruised and in extreme pain from the resuscitation itself, and she asked Mom not to allow that to happen again. "Don't let them resuscitate me anymore, Annie," she said. My mother saw to it.

A day or two later, Dad went to visit Grandma in the hospital. She said to him, "Come here." He went to her bedside. "Closer," she said. He leaned in. "Closer," she whispered, crooking a finger at him, and he bent down and put his ear by her mouth. In a loud, clear voice she shouted right into his ear, "Take me home!"

The doctors said that she had to stay where she was. "It was a different era," my father told me from his own deathbed. "We did what doctors told us back then." He paused. "She died in the hospital even though she asked me to bring her home. I'll never forgive myself."

THIRTY-NINE

Wheeling into Surgery

A hysterectomy is a common enough operation, but this is my first surgery, and I am attuned to every detail. While some women may experience this as routine, I am like an explorer in a foreign land, my newly acquired access both terrifying and fascinating.

The back of my bed is raised so that I am sitting almost upright as I'm wheeled from the little yellow, curtained "room" through a hallway, past a reception desk of some kind, and into the operating room. I've had to say goodbye to Craig and Mom. For a moment I'm bereft and afraid, and then I'm reminded, not unpleasantly, that we are all essentially alone, that every journey comes down to this moment, when only our eyes see what we experience, only we feel our hearts thumping, only we notice the green tile of the operating room and how enormous and bright the operating lights are. They look like bugs' eyes, with countless bulbs built to reflect the brightest light possible right up inside me, where no eyes or light have ever been, like the deepest darkest ocean cave—from utter darkness to blinding light. *This is my life*, I think, taking it all in. This is my life.

I am wide, wide awake, and a nurse leans into my face, smiling gently as she puts the back of my bed down so that I am lying flat. I smile back. She tells me her name. I don't remember it. There is a man in there too, fussing around. He has dark hair and is not the doctor. The nurse calls for the doctor on a phone, I guess, although I can't see her. Where is he, she wants to know. I can tell he's supposed to be there already, or maybe it's the anesthesiologist who's missing. I miss the anesthesiologist myself.

The guy with the dark hair and green scrubs who is fussing around is near my hand and I say, very quietly, "Hello," and although he's wearing a mask, I can see that he smiles at me with real warmth, as though he'd forgotten I was there and is so pleased to see me. He looks very busy but I can't help myself. "Will you hold my hand?" I ask him. He stops what he's doing and slips his gloved, but warm, hand into mine and pauses, and smiles again. He is better than anesthesia.

And then the anesthesiologist slams into the room, and the man in green scrubs drops my hand. "Sorry," says the anesthesiologist, sounding not really apologetic.

He asks me what I like to drink, and I tell him I like martinis. "Vodka?" he asks me.

"No, gin," I admit, although I don't mind vodka. He fills a syringe, or maybe it was already filled when he arrives. As he syringes it into my IV bag, he says, "Imagine this is Bombay Sapphire, then," bless his fucking heart. No kidding, even though I prefer Hendrick's.

By the time the word *Hendrick's* has gone across my synapses, the bright lights and green tiles and the smiling nurse and the fussing man with the warm hand are all quite disappeared.

FORTY

Happiness and Ostrich Feathers

When I was maybe twelve years old, my mother and I were driving across the Croton Dam near our home in Westchester, and she said to me, never taking her eyes from the road, "You can do whatever you want, you know. You can get married or not, or get married six times. You can have a thousand kids or no kids. You can be a lesbian or a nun, go to school, travel the world."

We drove for a while in silence while I sort of took in what she was saying, or tried to take it in. "The point is, all of the women who came before you would have killed to live right now. So be free. Do what you want. Be happy if you can." I'm still figuring out the implications of that conversation.

Grandma Hastings' Mardi Gras jewels were in a custom-built box in our attic when I was a child. The box looked like a baby's casket, and when my sister and I opened the lid, the fake emeralds and diamonds ("They're paste," Grandma had said, "but they're *good* paste, from Paris.") glittered dully in the light from the one naked attic light bulb. We were allowed to play with the crown, the scepter, the girdle of jewels that went around our waists, the ones that went around our wrists. We knew Grandma had been Queen of Rex, or that was a phrase we knew without understanding its import. Growing up in New York meant that Mardi Gras was just something we heard about on the news, a party where girls lifted their tops up for beads.

When I was thirty, I went to New Orleans alone and found that it was a big enough deal to have been Queen of Rex way back in 1911 that the Louisiana State Museum wanted those jewels from Mom's attic as well as the falling-apart mantle that Grandma had worn too. It was a big enough deal that the curator of textiles at the museum got a volunteer to spend over a hundred hours just on the mantle, reattaching ostrich plumes one feather at a time.

I will forever be an outsider to it all. Southern life remains a cipher to us Northerners. We are welcomed in to a certain extent but are rarely welcomed in all the way, and even then, Mardi Gras and the Rex organization have their secrets, *keep* their secrets. But here's what I do know. My great-great-grandmother, Mary Bella Brice, and great-great-grandfather, Judge A. G. Brice, raised Grandma Hastings after her young mother died of renal failure. Her father, feeling he was unable to raise the two young children in his charge, left them with their maternal grandparents. I know nothing about Grandma's brother, sadly. The judge, who always had a severe look on his face in photographs, was one of the behind-the-scenes organizers of Carnival in New Orleans in the 1800s. He and my great-great-grandmother, his wife, shunned publicity and kept a low profile, never wanting their names in the newspapers. But there had been an emergency. The woman slated to be Queen of Rex in 1911, Lois Janvier, had a death in the family and was expected to take a year of mourning. She most certainly could not reign as Queen of Mardi Gras that year, even though her dress had been fitted, the members of her court selected, the invitations sent. It was probably A. G. who decided, in that chaotic moment, to put his granddaughter Rose (Grandma Hastings to me) on the throne. There's no other way they would have condoned such ostentation.

There is only one photograph of her as Queen. She was nineteen years old, and beautiful, as all nineteen-year-olds are. In it, she sits on the throne bedecked in her jewels, resting her hand on her scepter, the same scepter I later held a thousand times. There the ostrich feathers that would one day disintegrate in my mother's attic frame her neck like a cloudlike collar. I wish I could ask her if she was shy to be photographed, or if she loved it, or simply felt it was another duty she had to perform. After all, she had been orphaned young and had been raised by her grandparents who were strict, educated, disciplined figures. Her life was filled with rules and duties, things to be carried out and overcome. A. G. Brice was the first mayor of Carrollton (a town in New Orleans), and a judge to boot. There was not a lot of room for whimsy in her life, I imagine. No one ever said to Rose, I bet, "Be free. Do what you want. Be happy if you can."

Within three years of her reign as queen, her fiancé and the love of her life would have killed himself, and within another fifteen years, the grandparents who had raised her would both be dead, she would have moved from New Orleans to New York, would have had two miscarriages and her week-old little girl, Mary, would have been born and buried in freezing, remote Constable, New York. But soon after little Mary died, she had my mother, and I hope, when I look at the picture of her as Queen of Rex, that eventually my mother's birth and survival were able to push Grandma's share of troubles off to one side.

This is where my childlessness hurts, when I think of what Grandma endured to have my mother, when I think of what she passed to me that I have nowhere to put. I feel her stories slip like sand through my open fingers and are blown away into nothingness. If I am not diligent, she will come to nothing, and it will be my fault.

FORTY-ONE

Just Post-Op

It is daylight, and I wake in a hospital room with a large window that looks out on the afternoon light and the autumn trees. Mom and Craig are there sitting by the window. They are there and I am alive. I am not back in my body yet but hovering over everything, waking back up to the present tense.

Dr. S is not there, but the younger one is, whom I've met at the office once or twice, who looks maybe thirty and very clean-cut, like he might have played sports in college, like he probably vacations on Martha's Vineyard and knows how to throw a spiral. I'll call him Dr. B, but I don't know if I ever learned his name. Dr. B knows I like medical stuff and that I can take him telling me what's really going on, so he says, "You lost a lot of blood during surgery." Oh. I think he says, "Five hundred milliliters," but I don't know how much that is really, or even if that's the number. "You are so healthy," he says. "Usually we see older women, or sicker women here, whose uterus is practically falling out, but yours didn't want to let go." He smiles. To some people this might be a bad bedside manner, but I like the way he is frank and informative, talking to me like he would talk to just about anyone. I don't think I say this out loud, but I definitely think, *Even in surgery I am a bleeder, I guess*.

"Because of the angle," he continues, "and the bleeding, Dr. S brought me and Dr. G in too, and we all decided together that he shouldn't bother with the second fallopian tube. He got the first one, but we all agreed that he should close, and since we were just removing them prophylactically, it was all right." I nod and smile. I understand. They took one fallopian tube and left the other. Got it.

"So you didn't have to go in abdominally, huh?"

"Nope." That is good news and means a quicker recovery of about a week. Great. Dr. B shows me with his hands about how big my uterus was and says that its size was unremarkable. In this case unremarkable is a good thing. "You have a catheter in so you won't have to get up tonight, but still, I'd like you to try to sit up. The sooner you can move your body around, the better."

They raise the back of my bed, and I have lots of little pings and explosions of pain in my rib cage. I grimace and the nurse says, "It's just air from the surgery," which I can't picture. And then I'm overcome by nausea and lie back down, sweating and panting. I hear my mother say to Craig, sotto voce, "She's so pale." I can feel that she is correct, like I am covered not in my skin but in the paper that encases garlic cloves or, better yet, tomatillos.

Things are beeping and a nurse is checking my urine output. The pillows they've put around my ankles whir and inflate, whir and deflate. I like them. It feels like I'm being hugged every minute or two. Night is falling, and I am in and out and don't care whether or not Mom and Craig stay. When they say they plan to go to a bar for a drink and to watch a game, I think it's a great idea. I have my own journey ahead, and I know I will need all my energy just to live it moment by moment.

I'm told that I will leave the next morning, "Barring anything unforeseen," says the young doctor. But the morning is so far away it's inconceivable. If it is now five or six in the evening, I have an entire twelve-plus hours left in the hospital, and that might as well be the width of the Atlantic with me doing the doggy paddle.

FORTY-TWO

Vivid Confusion

I ask for pain meds, but the nurse reminds me that taking a pill might increase my nausea. The air bubbles in my chest hurt, so I breathe into a spirometer or rather, I breathe *in*, pulling air *out* of the spirometer, and try to make that blue ball levitate. I have an insistent need to pee but I have a catheter in. The feeling of pressure on my bladder wakes me up over and over again. I call the nurse a few times and she checks the catheter, which is working. So why am I feeling so much pressure? Why won't my bladder relax and let me sleep? Sleep is tugging at me like a forceful undertow, and my bladder is tugging back.

As I lie in the hospital bed, I realize that I can probably have pain meds put in my IV drip. That shouldn't increase my nausea. When I ask, they say sure and they give me morphine (or something similar, I don't know) through my IV. As I drift off, I think about why I had to come up with that idea. *Why didn't they think of it?* I want to trust them, and this, like being asked my date of birth over and over again, is one of those hairline fractures that makes a spiderweb out of my trust.

There are lots of nurses of varying experience levels—some are young, like my college students, so thorough and not at all burned out yet. They urge me to drink my tea, my apple juice, my water, my milk. I try. I ask one to help me sit up. We try, she pushing at my back, me pulling on the arms of the bed, but the air bubbles in my chest hurt too much, so I give up and go back to sleep. My bladder is kicking at me with steel-toed cowboy boots even in my dreams.

The inflating pillows around my ankles whir and blow up, whir and deflate, circulating my blood so that I don't get clots. I continue to find them comforting, and in my twilight sleep—in addition to my bladder jabbing at me—the pillows make me think the cats are by my feet, turning in circles as they do before they settle in.

Later I watch five minutes of a black-and-white movie with Gregory Peck as a young priest. Is that a dream? I don't know. He is goddamned gorgeous, and that is not a dream. A new nurse comes in, older, a bit larger, and I think maybe she is strong enough to help me sit up. Sure enough she just sort of hauls me upright. I sit on the edge of my bed for a minute. A milestone.

Good. I slide back into bed and fall asleep, my bladder awake beside me mewling like an infant or a mosquito.

The night feels like it has no beginning or end, feels like I've been in it forever and will remain in it forever. Conversely, the night feels like a string of a billion single moments, mostly of pain, discomfort, and vivid confusion.

FORTY-THREE

Unpacking

It is dawn, and the sight of the trees outside my window and the blueing sky delight me. I have a forceful urge to be outside with what gives me joy—the smell of large stones, the quiet of forests. Even with my bladder throbbing, air bubbles beating against my rib cage, and a needle in the back of my hand, the trees and the sky outside my window are enough to remind me of why I love my life. Even if every single thing fell away from me, to stand under the quiet trees might be enough.

There is a little whiteboard in my room. It has places to fill in the following:

Today is: _____

Your nurse is: _____

Your patient care technician is: _____

Your rehab therapist is: _____

Today's goal: _____

The nurse manager is: _____

Most of the blanks are empty, but here's what has been filled in, using a blue marker.

Today is: Wed. 9/21

Your Nurse is: STACEY

In my mother's curly handwriting, a line has been added:

Your Praying Mantis is: CLAUDE

Today's goal: OUT OF BED!

I sit in my hospital bed, not laughing but grinning a lot.

THE YOUNG DOCTOR, Dr. B, comes in again. Has he been there all night? "I'll take the packing out now," he says. Because of the incision across the top wall of my vagina, where they removed my cervix and sliced through my vaginal wall, they have packed gauze into me, to apply pressure to this vascular-rich area and keep it from bleeding.

The way that Dr. B approaches this makes it seem like it will be nothing. A young nurse stands to my left. Dr. B pulls down the blanket, has me bend my knees, reaches between my legs and begins pulling out brown, bloodied gauze.

It hurts. It hurts a lot, actually, more than the bubbles in my chest, more than anything I can think of. In fact . . . OW!

His hands move fast, and I am groaning. He introduced this to me so casually. Hand over hand he pulls, like a sailor bringing in rope. Good lord! I finally say, "Stop," and seeing that I am grasping the nurse's hand with force, I ask her, "Did I hurt you?" "No," she says, smiling shyly.

"How much more is in there?" I ask the doctor.

"We're about halfway done." Jesus.

I hold the nurse's hand again. "Squeeze as hard as you'd like," she says, leaning in to my ear. She looks like she is eleven. Seriously. I'm reminded that nurses are angels in scrubs. I think briefly about my college writing students who are in the nursing program where I teach, and I am glad right now that their professors are so strict.

The doctor bends down and reaches back into me, and hand over hand, now reminding me of a magician pulling colored scarves out of his mouth, he pulls and pulls and pulls, while I groan and squeeze Brittany's hand (I think that was her name). In the end there is a pile of bloodied gauze on the bed between my legs. I am reminded, perversely, of the spaghetti scene in *Lady and the Tramp*.

"Holy shit," I say, because there really is no point in standing on ceremony when a guy has pulled a laundry basket of bloody rags out of your vagina, and you've practically broken a young nurse's hand.

When the doctor leaves, "Brittany" says to me, "I've never seen an unpacking before, and I'm really glad I was here for this. Now I know why my patients are so uncomfortable overnight." And now I know why I couldn't sleep. It wasn't the catheter. My bladder was being squished by this extraordinary amount of material packed into me. Again, with all of my affection for everyone here, couldn't they have told me about that yesterday? Couldn't they have said that, despite the catheter, I would feel as though I'd have to pee all night long, and not to worry?

For all I know, they did tell me, now that I think of it. There's a lot I don't remember. OK, I will give them the benefit of the doubt.

I sleep some more and drink my entire cup of tea. I eat a few bites of Farina because they are urging me to eat, and I drink the small fake orange juice (yuck) and breathe dutifully into (or, rather, out of) my spirometer.

I want to be well and go home. I'll do whatever they tell me to do. Home beckons.

Dr. B comes back in and takes out the catheter. I thought that would hurt, the removal of the catheter, but it doesn't. He unhooks the inflating pillows around my ankles, the ones that made me dream the cats were with me all night, adjusting themselves around my feet. "Let's get you up," he says, and with a nurse behind me and the doctor in front pulling on my arms, they basically lift me up to standing, yanking me straight through the pain of the air bubbles in my chest, and I am standing. Another milestone. Yay.

By the time Mom and Craig arrive, I am sitting in a chair with a blanket over me. They help me get back into my dress and flip-flops. The nurse sneaks me a few big absorbent sheets that I can put in my bed at home should I start to bleed a little, which they say is normal, and I get in a wheelchair where I am pushed to the parking lot, and then head for our house. I leave the hospital sure that within one week, two max, I'll be up and in decent shape, and I can get on with my life.

FORTY-FOUR

Mothers and Daughters

A few years ago when my mother came to visit, we sat in the sunroom one night, and she started telling me a story in the middle, as one does. "The phone rang in the dark of night," my mother said, "and I answered it. A woman's voice said 'Hello' and I said, 'Who is this?' and the woman paused and then said, 'It's your mother, downstairs.' She had her own phone line. Duh. 'I'm not feeling very well,' she said to me, so I went down and made her a cup of tea," my mother said, "and while the water was heating up I snuck a cigarette in the living room. After she'd had her tea, she still wasn't feeling any better, so I called her doctor, who said to bring her in to his office on Route 9."

I love it when Mom thinks of a story that has been with her all these years but she never thought to share before. I leaned in and she continued. "The building was dark, and the doctor had to turn on the lights one by one. It was quiet and strange. He called my mother by her first name, Rose, and he had her undress and lie on a table under a sheet while he felt around and asked her questions, and then he began to get her ready for an EKG, I suppose, and he pulled the sheet back, and I remember being shocked because I had never seen my mother's naked body before, and not only that, but I was able to see, for the first time, the shocking scar that went from her navel to her pubis from her Caesarean when I'd been born (which I know is not how it's done now, but all I can tell you is that's what I saw). And I remember that the scar looked ropy and gray in the fluorescent light.

"She was eighty years old and perfectly lucid, and the doctor just kept chatting with her and I finally said to my mother, 'Would you like me to cover you up?' and she said, 'Well, that would be very nice, Annie,' and so I pulled the sheet up to her neck.

"I suppose I remember that for two reasons. First of all, it was kind of comical that I didn't recognize my own mother's voice from downstairs on the phone. But it's also the shock of seeing her naked that burned it into my memory, and that scar, and how cold I thought she was, poor thing. But the scar and her nakedness." Mom paused. "And now I'm older than she was then." She paused again. "And I guess you're older now than I was then." Mothers and daughters.

Part Four

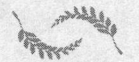

Home Again

FORTY-FIVE

Going Home

Getting from the hospital to our house feels outside of time. Every part of the journey is fractionated. I don't make one single trip home from the hospital. No, it's a thousand second-long journeys. I get from the wheelchair into the car. Then it's the car ride on the highway, where I hold my body so that it doesn't sway as we go around turns or get shaken when we thump over potholes.

Then it's our road.

Then our driveway.

Then our house, each segment separate, distinct, endured.

Our house. My heart is jumping (in a low-iron way) to see our house. From the car I can glimpse the zinnias still blooming to the side, yellow cucumber flowers still coming on, the mint a foot high and gone to flower.

The walk from the car to the front door is many minced steps, each its own day with its own orbit around a star. Arms on either side hold my elbows, half lifting me up the two front steps.

Inside the front door, the smell of boiled coffee, of cooking soup with rosemary in it, of sunshine baking the curtains.

Then there is the walk through the kitchen to the sunroom, normally six strides, but today seconds are like taffy, and this is a journey of endless strung-together seconds.

Now into the daybed—nice and high with clean sheets.

Craig helps me up into it and lowers me to horizontal.

Mom pulls up the blanket around my neck and tucks it around me so no air can get in or out.

My eyes flutter closed.

The sounds of the house, the pouring of the coffee, the meow of a hungry cat, my two most important people whispering to one another about me, I suspect. What they say doesn't matter. I am home.

There is nothing for me to do but *sleeeeep*.

FORTY-SIX

Coffee in an Egg Cup

By the time I've been home for a few hours, Mom and I have established our whole routine, which is one in a series of many routines we've established together over my lifetime.

Mom has turned from carefree companion to nurse. She's begun a list of pills that I've taken, and it sits by the kitchen sink with pill bottles lined up next to it: iron pills, stool softener, Percocet, ibuprofen. When any of us were sick as kids, she'd get out the fine dishes from New Orleans, the stuff that had belonged to Great-Great-Grandmother Brice, tiny dishes hand-painted with butterflies and flowers, all of which are now in the Louisiana State Museum. Mom would serve us ginger ale in handblown drinking glasses from the 1800s with initials etched on them. She had a way of making it so that every bit of contact you had when you were sick was filled with playfulness and beauty.

She's rummaged around my kitchen and found tiny bowls for my organic applesauce, and a few wee silver spoons that I bought at a yard sale. She's polished them, reminding me that when a person is focused on what matters, there is time for everything. This is the first polishing those spoons have had since they came home with me in a ziplock bag four or five summers ago.

I notice that she's moved her pillow to the other end of her futon bed so that her head will be closer to mine when we sleep. I am in and out, but try to notice, and realize even then how much of her I am not taking in. Her blond-white hair is still curled under. She seems perfect to me. When I ask for coffee, she brings it to me in the only piece of Great-Great-Grandmother Brice crockery that I own—a tiny egg cup. It is the perfect, adorable amount. I'm a fifty-something-year-old Stuart Little. This is how Mom rolls.

As NIGHT FALLS that first night home, and I am moving almost not at all, Mom goes through the CDs I put out before surgery and chooses Bach's cello adagios, which vibrate through my ribs in a pleasing way, like they are helping to knit me back together. I don't sit up, so I feel the bass notes in the mattress beneath me.

On the wall by my bed are the traced hands.

The cats, who have avoided the daybed because it is so high, pace back and forth on the floor beneath, and finally Zonker jumps up by my feet. Normally he would come up near my head and yowl for a face rub. Somehow he knows I can't pet him right now. Somehow he knows to stay by my feet. He curls up near them but not on them, such a little Buddhist monk, knowing just what is needed and what would be too much. He plants himself near me now and will not leave my side for weeks.

Claude is in the jade plant, hanging from his sticky feet. Mom reports his whereabouts to me. "He is on the move," she'll say, or "Good god, I don't know where he is," or "Yikes, I just found him hanging from the ceiling!"

The cello music and the warm purring cats, the praying mantis, my bed, all accumulate. There are living things all around me, and I am one of them, one of the living things.

It is time to sleep for the night, so that my body, which has been cut wide open, which has bled for all these months, and been anesthetized and sewn and medicated, can work its magic and reconstruct itself. I sleep and sleep and sleep, my feet warm, my mother nearby softly saying good night. It is my first twelve hours at home, but because I can only notice the most immediate things, it feels as though I have been home for a lifetime already, and with Mom there, as though this has been my only home since forever.

My thinking is that I will be the best patient on earth so that soon, in a day or two or three, I will be able to not be a patient anymore. I picture myself springing back into life, so much better than I was pre-op. I can see friends again. I can find a job. I can leave the house. So I rest, like the dutiful, determined patient that I am. I rest.

FORTY-SEVEN

A Bed of Polar Bears

The first few days after surgery swim together. There is nonspecific pain and bleeding. Some bleeding is expected, but this might be more than expected. I'm confused.

There is uncertainty, befuddlement. And shivering . . . a lot of shivering.

I am taking great big gulps of sleep like a thirsty person at a spigot. I sleep and sleep and sleep, ten, twelve, fourteen hours in a row, Zonker the one-eyed cat by my feet for all of it. When I shift, he shifts. He never touches me but is there. If I move my foot just so, I can feel his warmth through the blanket.

Whether I sleep for four minutes or four hours, there is Zonker.

ONE NIGHT THERE is a moon streaming in the sunroom windows onto my bed and I dream.

Zonker and I are sleeping on a bed of polar bears, who are, in turn, asleep on a floating chunk of ice adrift in the ocean.

It is nighttime, and the moon is full and shining on us, and I can feel it through my closed eyelids. The nighttime and the full moon are true both in the dream and in real life.

The polar bears turn this way and that in their sleep, and Zonker and I are warmed by their fur from underneath, with the cold arctic air on top of us. We are warm and cozy in the cold.

We float through the water, and then I watch as a whale plunges up through the black waters. He is navy blue and up and up he comes. (I am by his side under the water watching.) He opens his mouth wide, and now I can see down into his mouth as though I am hanging in the sky. I see the full moon reflected in the water pooled at the back of his throat.

He leaps up into the night and swings his hinged jaws shut.

I am filled with joy to be near him, such joy in his propulsion into the sky and his plunge back into his dark ocean depths. Zonker and I float on our ice floe until it bumps softly against land, until we have arrived at a place where I talk to Dad in the moon, as though they are one entity, Dad and the moon.

"Am I going to die?" I ask him from our ice floe, my eyes still closed.

"No," he says, straightforward, unemotional, pragmatic. He says, "Listen to this," and out of the dark blue sky comes Bach's Cello Adagio no. 1, the one I can't stop listening to.

"Hear that?" Dad says from the glowing moon.

"Yes."

"That is the sound of how loved you are."

Ahhhhh. I snuggle into the writhing polar bears, and Zonker turns over in his sleep, reaching a paw out to rest on my arm.

"And see that?" Dad says. I open my eyes and look up at the universe.

The light from the moon is refracting off of a kajillion dust motes that are falling through the night sky. Dad says, "Those are the stories you have left to tell."

Yes, I think, closing my eyes again and settling back down. *I have stories left to tell.*

FORTY-EIGHT

Trumpet Music from Next Door

Jerusalem artichoke: a perennial sunflower (*Helianthus tuberosus*) of the U.S. and Canada widely cultivated for its tubers that are used as a vegetable and as a livestock feed

—Merriam-Webster Collegiate Dictionary Online

My brain is not yet crisp, not yet handling intricate, sustained thought, moving instead in five-minute increments of "I have to get to the bathroom" or "I must take a pill" or "Let's see if I can turn over." I have no desire to write or think about anything complex, even as I know I still have stories in me. I dream vividly, and that's the extent of it for now, although I am semiconsciously gathering details even as I'm sick, to tell this story one day. My creative mind is wrapped up in my dreams, or it tends toward nature, toward the Jerusalem artichokes that are eight feet tall and blooming outside my window this late September.

I lie in bed and watch the wind push them back and forth.

When I was a little kid, there was a man named Warren who taught us all how to make maple syrup, how to carve spiles out of elderberry branches, how to push the soft pith out of their middles, hammer them into the tree's bark, and how to hang buckets there to catch the drops of welling-up maple water. I picture Warren's lanky frame chopping wood to boil the hauled sap into syrup, can see his ax in the air with the sun glinting off its blade, and the noise the ax made when it hit and split the wood.

One summer he ran a camp for us local kids where we built a garden together. He showed us how to grow Jerusalem artichokes, and later he dug up one of the roots, wiped the dirt off it with his thumb, and sliced it up for all the campers to eat. It was crisp like an apple slice, and a little sweet too, and still had some of the garden dirt on it. I think about him as I lie in bed staring at the sunflower-like blossoms, tall and quiet just like Warren was.

I think about the cats, the praying mantis still with us in the sunroom. There is a heartbeat to the natural world that is more fathomable than the world we humans construct. I'm not interested in the news, not interested in my computer or phone. I am completely absorbed by the thickness of the Jerusalem artichoke stalks, which seem able to withstand the power of the wind that blows around them, causing them to bend and sway but never break.

There is something about living in the suburbs of New Jersey that makes me long for weirdos. When I am in New Orleans (which is as often as I can arrange it), I feel as though I am home. In New Jersey, I always feel like I'm the one who doesn't fit in, whereas in New Orleans, I can relax. In New Orleans, I've seen aging socialites wear fur in summer to the grocery store. There are young guys there with thick black eyeliner who play the ukulele on the sidewalk, tracks up and down their arms, singing their guts out. One has a tiny dog on a leash. Another is wearing a porkpie hat and plays the harmonica badly, asking for money. I'd like to sit down in that folding chair near them and hold the guy's tiny dog. These are people I'd like to hang out with.

I don't get to see these people in the suburbs of New Jersey much . . . OK, ever. People like to fit in here. It's why I love the unseen guy who plays the trumpet around cocktail time every night. Is he next door with the chicken lady? Who can tell for sure? He plays the same tuneless song over and over again, every day, kind of scales but not that organized. The ludicrousness of it is heaven, makes me feel I am in the French Quarter for a minute.

I am not yet ready to think much about myself, and when I do, I'm not sure what to think anyway, so I listen to Bach, and to the trumpet music. I think of the mallards who have left already, and will one day return to the pond, I hope. I think of the feral cat out there, feeling the same wind that sways the plants in my garden. I daydream about standing once again in the woods, of feeling the wind on my skin and seeing what is out there.

FORTY-NINE

Silvano's Garden

A low hemoglobin count is generally defined as less than 13.5 grams of hemoglobin per deciliter (135 grams per liter) of blood for men, and less than 12 grams per deciliter (120 grams per liter) for women.

—Mayoclinic.org

Mom has moved two chairs out to the lawn. She's in her eighties and in excellent shape. She never stops moving, even if she is a bit slower on stairs than she used to be. "My shoulder isn't great," she says, which I know because I can hear her in the kitchen asking Craig to reach her things that are on the upper shelves. "Can you get that coffee cup for me?" "Can you reach me the paprika?" She is also bossy, in general. She knows how things ought to be, and if she can't make them that way herself, she speaks the hell up, quietly, genteelly, with that curled-under hair. She doesn't settle.

I settle all the time. I want to be more like her, and I picture the way Grandma Hastings used to make Wheatena (or was it Cream of Wheat?) every morning when she lived with us. She'd stand at the stove and stir. There is something about her certainty of how things ought to be that lives on in Mom but missed me. I've never had the same breakfast two days in a row. I've never done anything two days in a row.

Craig has gone off to work, and I've watched Mom move the two chairs out to the lawn by herself. I go out there with my walking stick. We sit under the maple tree. Before work Craig went to the deli down the road and got her the paper (as he'll do every morning for her). She reads the paper and I read poems. People have sent me books and books and books, so I read W. B. Yeats and Mary Oliver. Poems are perfect for healing—tiny bites of squished language, designed it seems for the way that healing feels finely delineated and intense and compressed. The chair and the walking stick. The cardinal at the feeder. The funny ache in my gut with no visible injury, other than the mark the tape left when they removed my IV way back during the D&C. The deep, deep-in-my-bones exhaustion. I'm newly aware of all the muscles and energy needed just to hold my head up, so I sit outside for five whole minutes and then begin the trip back inside to get horizontal.

I am preoccupied with bodily functions. My hemoglobin levels have been low (hovering just around 7) since before the operation, and although I haven't been to the doctor yet since surgery, I can sense that they are still low. I've lost so much blood for so long, but I don't want to take iron pills because they will constipate me. It feels important to facilitate my body's elimination of waste, and if I have to choose between low hemoglobin levels and excretion, excretion seems more fundamental and urgent. So we look up what foods will boost my iron levels, and Mom goes to the store (driven by Craig) and buys lentils, ground beef, and leafy greens.

On Saturday she and Craig pay a visit to our friends Mary and Silvano. They are in their eighties and have the most bountiful garden on their single acre: over a hundred tomato plants, a fig tree, a tunnel covered in melon vines and milk pumpkins for fall pies. Silvano sends Mom home with thick branches of rosemary and stalks of thin, fibrous, dark green celery topped with enormous leaves. Mom sets about making me a celery broth (from my daybed, I can hear her chopping for what seems like hours, *chop chop chop*).

The smell in the house from Mom cooking does something to me. I become quite totally awake and newly ravenous. Mom gets me upright and sitting on a chair in the kitchen. She hands me a tiny bowl of broth. I hold it, warm in my hands like a little bird just tipped out of its nest. *Sip sip sip.* I don't have the energy to speak, but I want more, right now, so I hold the bowl out and Mom refills it. *Sip sip sip.* The more I drink the more I want. I've never tasted anything like it, warm, soft, slightly salty. It soothes my throat and warms my chest, and I can feel my body crying out for more. More. More.

After four tiny bowls of hot celery broth, my body is euphoric, my belly full of what feels like the sea. I make it the six or so steps back to the bed in the sunroom. Someone helps me lie down, feeling like Silvano's garden is growing inside of me. I don't remember the covers being pulled up, but they are. I don't remember Zonker joining me, but he does.

FIFTY

Mom's Celery Broth Recipe

Mom sent me the following recipe via email once she had gone home.

MOM'S CELERY BROTH RECIPE

If you are lucky enough to have a farmer nearby, or a farm stand that is selling locally grown celery, by all means use their product: it's fresher and more pungent, more flavorful than what comes packaged in a store.

SERVES 2 IN SMALL SOUP BOWLS

5 long stalks of dark green outer celery, cut up very small. You may find that you can pull off some of the fibrous "strings" from the stalks and discard them.

10 to 12 sprigs of Italian parsley. Cut leaves from stems and chop them up.

Add the celery and parsley to a pot holding 3 cups of chicken broth or bone broth or just plain water.

Lay one sprig of rosemary atop. The "needles" will soften and fall off and the stem can be discarded before serving.

Boil with lid on for about half an hour (or more depending on how soft you want the celery). Check every so often to see that you have enough water. Add more if needed.

I added no seasoning because this was for someone feeling queasy with no real appetite, and I wanted it to be bland yet tasty and restorative.

FIFTY-ONE

Wheatena

When Grandma Hastings stood at our stove in the mornings stirring her Wheatena, she'd cut up two or three prunes in it. This was her morning ritual. She used the same little copper-bottomed pot each time and the same wooden spoon, and she'd stand, with her long gray hair coiled up in a tight bun, and stir and stir until it was ready. Then she'd tip it into a bowl and wash the pot and wooden spoon before she sat down at the breakfast room table to eat.

I think of her neat bun, of her long skirts, of her wooden spoon and tidiness, of her certainty over the right thing to eat, the right thing to do, day after day after day. Such discipline. It's a wonder to me, that kind of steadfastness. There are small things that happen in front of us and how are we to predict how they will influence us?

Mom still has that little pot with the copper bottom. Mom still has that wooden spoon, its edges softened by decades of stirring.

FIFTY-TWO

The Volume of the World

Recovery after vaginal hysterectomy is shorter and less painful than it is after an abdominal hysterectomy. A full recovery might take three to four weeks.

Even if you feel recovered, don't lift anything heavy—more than 20 pounds (9.1 kilograms)—or have vaginal intercourse until six weeks after surgery.

—MayoClinic.org

I'm five days out from surgery, and I am still sleeping a lot, but I feel like I'm on track, like I am doing and experiencing exactly what was predicted.

The volume of the world is dialed way down.

I am intimate with the sound of my heartbeat against the pillow, with the swelling of my left hand where they slid in, then removed, an IV needle. The black-and-blue stain there recedes slowly, like the most lugubrious of outgoing tides. I watch it. I touch it to see if it's tender, its healing a kind of barometer for my overall healing.

I see Claude hanging from Mom's cobalt-blue stained-glass window that hangs in the sunroom. Years ago, when I was a kid, Mom drove past a bank that was being torn down and found a stack of arched windows on the sidewalk waiting to be carted to the dump. "It's oak," she tells me now, "so it weighs a ton. I should have taken them all, but I could only get two into my car." Mom is an artist. For some reason I contemplate what it will be like having that window hanging here long after Mom will one day be gone. It's a sad and comforting thought.

I wear a coat and sit in a chair outside, my mother in a chair nearby, both of us reading. She is really reading, while I pick up my Yeats from time to time and read a line, and then put the book down and close my eyes.

She is eighty-three and I am fifty-two. She is the person on earth who most wants me alive, my friend for fifty-two years. We don't have to talk. But we do. From time to time.

All of the presurgery anxiety and jitteriness is vanished. I move slowly. My eyes don't even try to see far away. I do not think of cell phones. I do not think of elections. Bank accounts do not occur to me. Such pleasure to float above the matters of the earth and of industry.

The world has shrunk down and down and blessedly down to just our lawn filled with maple tree seed pods, which crackle beneath my shoes and the rubber tip of my walking stick as I make my way back inside and into bed.

FIFTY-THREE

Shivering

How many days have gone by? I don't know really, except that I started writing poems five days after I got home and thought, "Five days is how long it takes to heal enough to write a poem."

I've made other kinds of progress in addition to poem writing. I walked to the first turn in the driveway. And then later I walked to the bottom of the driveway and back up. And then all the way to the bottom of the driveway and just beyond to the mailbox. I'm feeling stronger, opening the packages that have come in the mail. The outpouring continues. There are friends who haven't called at all, and others who have visited with ice cream. All of it is welcome, even the ones who don't call. It's all just how it's supposed to be.

When I was in sixth grade, I was stuck at home with mono for a whole month. Every day, when my dad went to work, he sent me a postcard from his job in New York City. All of the boxes and cards now remind me of

Dad, and of being in sixth grade when life felt so hard I sometimes wondered if I'd make it through alive. What I'm going through now is much easier than sixth grade, I remind myself. Everything on earth is much easier than sixth grade.

I continue to use the walking stick as a cane and have not yet gone upstairs. The bathroom remains an issue. There is pain and a little blood on the pads I keep wearing. I've taken only one Percocet because I don't want to get constipated. I've decided to save the rest for a time (much later, and hopefully never) when I might wish I had a stockpile.

I continue to lean on the ibuprofen, the big ones, prescription strength. When I haven't had one, it's not pain that gets to me but shivering. Postsurgical pain is usually just incisional, and with the vagina being so sensitive in some ways, how is it that the incision there is entirely devoid of sensation for me now? The nerve endings in organs, as I understand it, don't provide the kind of discrete sensory information that the nerve endings in, say, your eyes or fingertips do. Although the painful menstrual cramps I used to experience tell me there must have been nerve endings in the muscles of my uterus. They're gone now. At any rate, I take the ibuprofen not because of specific pain but because, without it, I get so cold that I shake and shake and shake and begin to cry, although I have nothing to cry about. I weep and get to bed and shiver under the covers. The shivering is exhausting. I imagine that the shivering is my body's way of telling me to lie down and rest, the way pain would normally instruct me to do, so I listen to it. And it feels a little bit like pain, if discomfort and confusion were construed as pain.

For this reason, I stay up on the ibuprofen. I am supposed to take one every six hours. Mom makes note of when I last took one, and I try to make sure that I don't go beyond the six hours. If I keep a rather steady stream of it in me, I'm fine. If I let too many hours go by, say nine hours instead of six, I take a pill and it can be a full hour after that when the shivering finally stops. I stop trying to be brave and just take the pills to help my body heal.

FIFTY-FOUR

Learning to Read

When Grandma Hastings came to live with us, I couldn't yet read, despite being read to every night before bed. She cut up some vellum and folded it into a tiny book, first sewing the spine with a needle and thread, then tying the spine with a silky blue ribbon. She wrote *Nanette Reads* on the cover, and inside she would write a sentence or two, "See the bee. I like the bee," for example, and I would illustrate it in my five-year-old way. Grandma Hastings very patiently taught me to read.

She taught me to read.

I miss her so forcefully. She died that year but not before she taught me to read. I see her in that house, which was brimming with cats and dogs and children, brimming with musical instruments and lacrosse sticks and macramé beads. She has the picture of a dove with an olive branch in its mouth pinned to her door, and I am allowed inside. In that room is an adult who is not rushing anywhere. She wants to be needed, and I am little and full of need. Inside that room is an adult who is pleased to have quiet time with me. Inside that room is this woman who loves me and is going to co-write my first little vellum book with me. She is going to help me fall asleep at night. She is going to teach me to read.

I'm holding the book she made for me in my hands right now and see for the first time that there is a ring from a coffee cup on the back cover. I run my finger around the circle and think that maybe that was from Grandma Hastings' very own coffee cup.

The book is half empty. The last sentences she wrote were, "Eat the cake. Sweet cake." I never made an illustration for that page. I suspect that when Grandma died, Mom just packed the little book into a box in the attic where I would find it almost fifty years later, and left the little blue ribbon that had come undone for me to retie.

FIFTY-FIVE

In Another Room

As I begin to pull out of the fog, I realize that Craig is not so present in all of this. It's much more me and Mom, which is fine, actually, but I'm aware of it. Craig and I have been married for over a decade, together a few years longer than that. He's quiet. I'm effusive. But we sleep in a small bed, and our arms are always around one another. It's like taking a vitamin, living with him.

He's a weirdo too. I mean, he will not order what anyone else orders when we go to a restaurant. It doesn't matter how much he wants the eggplant Parmesan, he won't order it if anyone at our table chooses it first. And he sings, not around people, but in his sleep (when he's especially happy), or in the shower. They're made-up songs he sings. He's in the shower right now and singing something about the hike he's going on later. "It's going to be a great day," he'll sing. When he goes to church, he multiplies one hymn number by another in his head. We really couldn't be less alike.

While I'm sick, though, and while Mom is in the house, he is never completely himself. We don't get to whisper and laugh in bed the way we normally do once the lights are off. There's none of that now. We're in separate rooms, on separate floors of the house. Normally, when he watches football, I bring a book and lie on the couch with him, our heads on opposite ends, and read. There is none of that now either.

The women are in the sunroom dealing with blood, with healing, our own quiet whisperings in the night. It feels old-fashioned, being separated from him, but it also feels correct. He is nearby, and that comforts me. Mom is with me, and I imagine that comforts Craig, gives him leave to do whatever it is that he does when I'm not around.

CRAIG IS ALSO busy with work, and I'm aware of his subtly lowered rank while Mom is in the house. He wakes up early, gets Mom her newspaper, heads off to fight New Jersey traffic on his way into work. When he arrives home at night, I hear Mom ask him for things. "Reach me the tin foil, would you?" she'll ask the minute he comes in the door, and "Where do you keep the olive oil?" or "How do I turn on the oven?" Then there are the lists she hands him. "We need to get gauze and chamomile tea and more ibuprofen." I want to tell her to knock it off with the lists, that he just got home from work, but I am in another room (in more ways than one), and I cannot expend that kind of energy. They will work it out. I listen from my bed, in and out of sleep, trusting that soon it will be just Craig and me again.

One afternoon while Mom is taking a nap, Craig sneaks in to say hello. We smile into each other's faces. I tell him that I'm sorry we're not together. "Don't worry. We're barnacles," he says, "stuck together on a ship for life."

FIFTY-SIX

A Question for Mom

Mom and I have now spent just over a week together, twenty-four hours a day. We have lists of pills I've taken, lists of food I've eaten, sleeping details, bowel movement information. It's pretty sexy stuff. My calendar is full of upcoming doctor appointments and reminders. She has a shopping list on the counter. It is as though she is instructing me, or reminding me, of simple things that she taught me a long time ago: Keep the sink empty. Eat fresh food. Find patches of sun and sit in them. Slow down. Be content. It is like reviewing lessons from childhood about how to take care of myself, and I love it. I'd forgotten all of it.

We don't talk much. She reads all of *Harriet the Spy* to me. It's one of my favorite books from childhood, a book Dad gave me, and Mom has never read it. I cry when she reads Ole Golly's letter to Harriet, just as I did way back in first grade when I read it alone. She gets a little misty too.

From time to time, we pick up the Yeats and read to one another, or we read from the Robert Louis Stevenson book she brought with her (god, he's dated). It is these long swaths of time together that are blessed intimacy. We are old friends, she and I. She feels more like my sister now than my mother. I am aware that she moves through the world with such humor and care. I am still learning from her, not only how to take care of myself and how to keep a kitchen clean. She also teaches me how to have enough time to watch the birds. She always has enough time. It is obvious every second how lucky I am to have her here with me, not just now, but especially now.

In some ways I married my mother when I married Craig. The two of them are happy, kind, even-tempered. I say about Craig, "If I am a balloon, then he's the guy holding the string." He keeps me from floating off into late night worries.

Still, they're different from one another too. When Craig gets home after work, he brings a livelier, messier energy with him. He crashes in the front door shouting, "I'm home!" The cats get up to greet him, hoping for wet food. He brings in the mail and groceries, has news of the outside world. He figures out if there's a movie for the three of us to watch, and he wants to know how our day has been, and behind him, in a great swath of abundance, he leaves mail on counters, cabinet doors flung open, and a trail of pennies and nickels that seem to fall from his pockets wherever he walks or sits. Normally I can cope with this, but I am dimly aware of not being well enough to follow behind him and gather up the mail or close the cabinet doors, and that it is left to Mom. I figure I won't be able to keep things together after she's gone home for long.

But the daytimes are quiet, Mom and I never more than a few feet away from one another. There is never a dirty dish in the sink while Mom is there, which is an enormous pleasure to me.

And it is on one of the chilly late-September afternoons, as we are sitting in a patch of sunlight in the yard, seven or eight or nine days after surgery, that I say, "You have been a role model for so many things: how to have a happy marriage, how to run a household, how to grow older. Your old age has been so active with all of us kids, just as Grandma Hastings' old age was taken up with you and your children. You take an interest in everything we do. Here you are taking care of me. But because I don't have kids and you do, I am not sure how to live a happy old age without children. How do you think you would manage to be happy at this stage of life if you didn't have any children?"

We sit there in silence. She puts her paper on her lap and stares into the middle distance. "Jesus," she says. It's a big question, maybe a stupid question, maybe unanswerable.

"Forget it," I say. "It's an impossible question."

"No," she says, "but I need time. I need to think it over."

FIFTY-SEVEN

Mantids in Winter

I've started watching the news a little bit. I only remember this because I make note of something then New Jersey Governor Christie says that annoys me. He says that a train out of Hoboken was "traveling at a high rate of speed." Why can't he just say: "traveling at a high speed" or "going too fast"? Hmmm. The editing part of my brain must have reawakened.

I have read over the ten or so xeroxed pages that the hospital sent home with me. They are full of instructions, what to expect, warnings, phone numbers to call in an emergency, but deciding what is an emergency is fuzzy. Everything sort of sucks, but nothing is truly emergent.

The ten pages are about constipation, about vaginal discharge, about insurance, and pain killers. It's a lot of pages that don't say much, and that feel more like a bureaucracy's defense against litigation than actual patient care. I can just picture a room full of VPs voting on the packet's contents, and some bald guy in a gray suit, his left eye twitching, saying, "Legal wants us to make sure to say 'persons' instead of 'people.'"

If I were to write the manual for being at home just after surgery, I would say, "Your body is different now. Sit quietly and listen to it." I would say, "You're afraid, I bet, but so is everyone." I would say, "Every second, your entire body is rallying to your defense."

I would say, "Get through the next minute . . . and then get through the minute after that." Legal would never go for any of it.

As September becomes October, I can feel the cold, and I worry about what will happen to Claude, who is, even now, in the Christmas cactus. I should ask Craig to carry that Christmas cactus inside the house proper soon. I can't carry it yet, but we can't move it anyway, not if Claude is on it. I don't think he can live inside (not that I particularly want him in the house). But I don't think mantids live through the winter.

Perhaps, one day soon I'll have the energy to google the life cycle of a praying mantis, but not today. Not just yet.

FIFTY-EIGHT

Cocktail Time: A Setback

Suddenly it's time for Mom to leave. She's been with me for over a week and a day now and her dentist appointment looms, so she will leave first thing in the morning. We sit in the sunroom at five, as we do every evening. Tonight, she makes herself a manhattan and serves me one of my cold-pressed juices in a wineglass. She makes a little plate of something beautiful for us to share—ripe pear slices with Brie and a pile of arugula with cherry tomatoes to eat with our fingers.

My ibuprofen wore off an hour ago and I'm beginning to shiver when I take a piece of ice-cold pear with Brie in my fingers. I eat it. It tastes like perfume—gorgeous. I want more but I start to cry.

"What's wrong?"

I'm laughing and crying at the same time, knowing how ridiculous this is. I'm full-on sobbing. "The pear is so cold on my fingertips," I'm wailing. What is wrong with me? "I can't pick it up. It's too cold." I'm weeping.

She laughs at me and gets me an ibuprofen and my scarf. I'm already wearing a coat.

I suddenly feel wetness under me and push up to almost standing. I have bled through the pad I'm wearing and all over the seat cushion. It is the bright red of fresh blood. It is a lot of blood. My crying stops, as it does when things are actually bad. There's no room for that now. I need to get to the bathroom, need to change, need to warm up, need to figure out why I am bleeding. And of course, it's after five and no doctor will answer the phone. And Mom has to leave in the morning.

We start to keep track of how many pads I will go through during the night. I'm not supposed to be bleeding like this. It's the kind of thing that could maybe rcsolve itself, but it's so much blood that I am privately worried that I might have to go to the emergency room if it increases even a little. I go through five maxi pads that night. I do not sleep.

In the morning the bleeding has slowed, and Mom has to leave. I walk her out to my sister's boyfriend's car (he's come to pick her up). I lean on my cane, stand in the driveway, smiling and waving. I walk to the top of our stone steps and smile and wave at the back of the car that is taking her away. It feels like my heartbeat is driving off without me.

Part Five

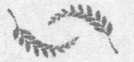

Relapse

FIFTY-NINE

Matzo Brei and the Color of Blood

Because it is chilly now, Craig and his friend move the daybed indoors from the sunroom for me. For two days I fend for myself . . . keep my own list of meds. I cook. I am alone all day, and Craig brings home groceries after work. He washes the dishes. I can't climb the stairs yet, so he stays downstairs nearby, sleeps on the couch where I can hear him breathe. My barnacle.

I am not supposed to be bleeding like this, and I'm moving slowly, thinking slowly. Should I have called the doctor last night, or is this no big deal? I don't know. When I finally do call, I reach a woman I've never spoken to before. She is the doctor on call and doesn't know me, and she's clearly alarmed by what I'm describing. "You're not supposed to be bleeding, and you're not supposed to be bleeding like *that*!" My body feels achy and not right. I ask her if she thinks I should go to the emergency room. She hesitates. "Just get into the office now," she tells me.

Craig takes the morning off from work and brings me in for this first post-Mom doctor appointment. I can't tell if it's an emergency or not, but they do whisk me in the minute that I get there.

The office is small, and Craig has a legal pad for taking notes. He sits next to me on a little stool with wheels. I'm in the stirrups, and Dr. S peers inside me. "I'm going to call Dr. G in, OK?" Yes, but there won't be room for Craig. Dr. S is funny. He says to Craig, "You want to wheel into the little changing room there?" It's just a cut-out behind a curtain where I changed into my gown a few minutes earlier.

"Sure," says Craig. Dr. G comes in and then the young one, Dr. B, comes in too. All three of them bend over between my legs, peering, squinting inside me with headlamps on like a bunch of coal miners.

"What color was the blood?" Dr. G asks me.

"What do you mean?" I ask.

"Well, was it dark? Was it red or brown? Blackish maybe? Thick?"

"Who am I? Renoir?" I ask. They laugh. I love these guys. "It's red. Not thick like menstrual blood, thin and red. Not black. Maybe brown. I don't know."

Craig sticks his head out from behind the curtain and scares the crap out of the young one, Dr. B, who jumps and then says a warm, "Hey! Craig!" They're sort of friends because it turns out that Dr. B went to Fordham and Craig went to Notre Dame, bonding over their assumed Catholicism. Before I met Craig, I didn't know a thing about Notre Dame. Now I am amazed repeatedly at how his affiliation with them affords us friends everywhere. We were in Alaska, of all places, going to see a baseball game, and ended up in the near-empty stadium with a group of Notre Dame alums buying us beer. I graduated from Sarah Lawrence. I have literally never run into an alum from Sarah Lawrence, and if I did, I wouldn't know how to recognize them or what to do. Anyway.

The doctors are worried. The bleeding is getting more copious, if anything, and my hemoglobin levels are dipping ever lower. They want me to take iron pills, but I don't want to get constipated, don't want to have to strain because there are stiches inside me that could pull and cause even more bleeding. The doctors want to see me every day now, and Craig drives me to the doctor's office on his way to work, where I undress and get back into the stirrups.

I know it sounds ridiculous, but it's hard work for me to get dressed to go see the doctors, to get to the car, to get from the car to the doctors' office, and then from the office to the exam room. I am not well. I can tell, and so can the doctors. I feel like I'm fading. I am freezing always and worn out. I've started calling my walking stick a cane, and I use my cane all the time now.

I go to the doctor five times in one week. My hemoglobin levels won't rise, and every morning we all hope the bleeding will stop, that my body will heal whatever wound is open inside me, but it doesn't. We're weeks into recovery now and I am bleeding almost as much as I was before the surgery.

One day the doctors use a long Q-tip and apply a coagulant to the healing wound up inside me. I get home and there is no blood for an hour. I'm hopeful and tentative, and then the dam bursts. They order bedrest. They tell me not to pick up anything, even something light. They tell me not to climb the stairs. I do what I'm told.

The morning after the Q-tip, I go back in. Undress. Back in stirrups. It gets so that I am comfortable having a room full of men bending down between my legs and looking in there like I am a car with my hood up. I get so comfortable in fact that I feel like I could walk around the doctor's office half-naked and not feel self-conscious. This is unusual for me, who doesn't even like to shower naked, but we're all sort of friends, and who has the energy to care about such things? The fact that I make it back and forth to their office is kind of impressive, to me anyway.

We are so relaxed around one another that on one visit, I don't know why, maybe because Dr. S sounds so much like Grandma Moss, I sit in the stirrups, with the three of them gathering around craning their necks for a good view and I say to the ceiling, "When was the last time you had good matzo brei?"

Dr. G stands up, thinking. "Oh, years. It's been years."

Dr. S says, "Matzo brei? I haven't had that since I was a kid."

The young doctor, the Fordham gentile guy, says, "What's matzo brei?"

"It's the most boring food really," I say, "just scrambled eggs and matzo, a little salt maybe, but my grandmother used to make it. Very comforting. You could get it in diners when I was a kid, but I haven't had any in years, and now I'm craving it." With me still in the stirrups, Dr. G gets his phone out of his white coat and googles matzo brei, and shows it to the young Fordham doctor, who shrugs.

"It doesn't look like much," says Dr. G. "You have to try it."

"My grandmother sometimes put onions in," I say.

"Fancy," says Dr. S, who hasn't stopped looking inside of me the whole time.

THE LONG AND short of it is, we have a problem. They keep hoping it will resolve itself, that the bleeding will stop, because if it doesn't, they'll have to open me back up to find out what's bleeding, and nobody wants that. Meanwhile I am weak—weak from the surgery, weak from the months of heavy bleeding leading up to the surgery, and newly weak from this new bout of unexpected bleeding. "Let's see if your body can stop the bleeding on its own," they tell me. "No lifting of *anything*." they repeat. "No driving. No sex. No housework. No stairs. Just rest. Just lie in bed and rest. The best thing would be if your body could heal itself."

Indeed. I refuse to even contemplate going back in for more surgery. Come on, I tell my body. Come on. We can do this.

I'M TOO TIRED to be upset, but I'm busy actively sleeping fourteen, sixteen hours at a clip, which is wildly unusual for me. Now in the morning, I lift my groggy head . . . Get dressed for the doctors . . . Rest . . . Brush

my teeth . . . Rest . . . Take my pills . . . Rest . . . Get to
the car . . . Sleep in the car . . . Get to the doctor . . . Be
completely still.

People in the waiting room are mad about things,
mad about having to wait for an appointment, mad
about I don't know what. I do not have the energy to be
mad. I do not have the energy to think about their anger.
I am just focusing on staying warm and upright until
they call me in. I want to lie down. I want to sleep. My
body is telling me to sleep. I am busy hoping that I am
not, right this very second, bleeding all over the couch in
the nice doctors' waiting room. There may be no energy
for anger, but there's always energy for a little shame.

SIXTY

Carving Camellias

A recording of Grandma Hastings has survived. Dad, who was on the radio and regularly interviewed celebrities, got out his reel-to-reel recorder in 1960 and conducted an interview with his mother-in-law. Craig digitized it, and I listen to it once in a while, maybe every two or three years. I like to hear her soft voice. I like to be reminded of her lovely New Orleans accent, to remember what she sounded like when I was a little girl in her bed, unable to sleep. I find it on my laptop. I want to hear her now.

They talk about the post-Reconstruction era in New Orleans, and how Grandma Hastings was raised by her grandparents, Mary Bella and Judge A. G. Brice, who had lived through the Civil War. It was, therefore, a very old-fashioned home she grew up in, and Grandma spoke about the strict rules that Mary Bella Brice (my great-great-grandmother and Grandma Hastings' de facto mother) imposed on the household.

"Well," I listen to Grandma say, "she wouldn't let you talk about sickness, and she wouldn't let you talk personalities. Oh, and talking about the war was barred, except in instances where it was discussed without feeling."

"What *could* you talk about?" I hear my father ask in the background.

"You could talk about history or plants or flowers or animals."

Such stringent rules probably made life easier for those left bruised by the Civil War, and from what I know of this long-dead great-great-grandmother of mine, she was a powerful woman who knew how to survive. By the time she was twenty-eight years old, her first husband had died along with two of her four children. I had forgotten that, but I hear it again and long for her presence with force.

Dad asks her about yellow fever. I've listened to this interview dozens of times, but I'd completely forgotten this episode, and it's like hearing it for the first time. She said, "There were two conditions down in New Orleans that caused the greatest fear . . . One was high water and the other was yellow fever." She was nine years old when she caught it in 1897.

"What happened when a household was stricken in that way, it was put under quarantine with the guards at our front and back door, and a yellow flag was tacked up on the gatepost so that everybody was warned. Later my brother came down with it too, and here were the guards at the front door and the back door. And only the doctor could come in and go out.

"Yellow fever was nothing to play with. It was a very dangerous and a very quick killer. Seems that Grandmother Brice had had a great deal of experience nursing yellow fever and had administered medicines and even organized a nursing service among the ladies who had escaped the disease.

"Well, anyway, here were Willie and I down with the yellow fever and nothing very much to do. The guards would entertain us by sending in carved vegetables. I remember the beautiful white turnips that were carved to look like camellias. It was delightful. I don't remember much about it except that I came out successfully. I don't even know how long I was sick. But anyway, Grandmother [Brice] did her usual good job of bringing us through what was a very deadly peril."

I'm struck again by the way grandmothers and mothers and daughters have cared for one another as long back as I can find records in my family. Maybe all families are like that, but it feels like an inheritance to hear Grandma again this time.

Listening to my beloved grandmother's voice does something similar to what listening to cello adagios does. It pieces me back together.

SIXTY-ONE

Mom Returns

My bleeding doesn't stop and the doctors are worried. I am also not able to crap comfortably. I'm shaky and frustrated. One night I soaked through several pads and then all over the mattress. I really thought this was all behind me, would all be behind me after the surgery. And this is worrisome, of course, because it's not coming from my uterus (which is gone, needless to say). Something is bleeding internally. I feel up to my ankles in blood. And I'm trying to eat iron-rich foods, but I find it hard to cook and clean and take care of myself. I keep thinking about how Mom kept the sink empty, but it is never empty now. Help!

I get out of bed and put a pan on the stove. I put oil in the pan and then my heart is racing and I am so exhausted that I have to lie down for ten minutes. I get up, turn on the burner and put the ground beef in the pan and stand stirring for a few minutes, but I have to lie down, so I turn it off again. Making a small meal, eating it, and cleaning up after it is taking me hours. I'm not even hungry, but my body needs iron, so I'm trying to keep up the level of care that my mother started for me, or even a fraction of that. And I'm taking these stool softeners because I am not supposed to strain for fear of popping internal sutures and causing yet more bleeding.

But one day I take too many stool softeners I guess, and Craig is at work, and Mom has gone home, and I am lying in bed and have an accident, or as my friend later calls it, a "poopsplosion." Well, that'll get you up and out of bed *fast*. I get to the bathroom and strip down, put all my clothes in the sink, start to clean myself off, and then I think of all I need to do in the next ten minutes. I'm freezing already, shaking. I am bleeding too and need to rinse my underwear and clothes a little before putting them in the washing machine. I need a new pad, and to go all the way upstairs (I'm not supposed to climb stairs, as per my doctor's orders, and I haven't climbed stairs since the surgery until now) to find clean clothes. I need to shower.

For a moment there in the kitchen, I have a soundless internal meltdown and then start to figure out how to proceed. *So let's prioritize*, I think. *What's most important?* Shivering won't kill me. I take a spoonful of (very cold) applesauce and swallow an ibuprofen and write it on the pad by the sink. I'm naked and I'm trembling cold, the floor is like ice, but it's triage and the medicine will be more important in the long run than cold feet, which will, eventually, get warm. I'm still naked when I find my phone and call Craig at work to ask if he can come home. I get his voicemail. I do everything slowly because I don't want to have to do anything twice, don't want to fall or further complicate things. It will take him an hour to get home if he can even leave work, if he even listens to this voicemail.

By the time he does get home, I am washed and dressed. (I literally crawled up the stairs for clean clothes.) I'm asleep in the daybed despite the mound of dishes in the sink, despite the crumbs of cat food on the floor by their dish. The laundry is washed and waiting to be put in the dryer. I have emailed Mom. "I hate to ask you this. I know you have so much to take care of in your own life, but I am sitting here in the kitchen shaking and bleeding like crazy. I don't have the energy to fix my own food. I can't remember when I took my medicine. Is there any way you can come back?" I send that email right after my shower, possibly before I think to call Craig. Two hours after Craig comes home from work, my mother pulls into the driveway, chauffeured by my sister's boyfriend. Everyone is pitching in.

I don't see my mother arrive. I just hear the sound of car tires rolling slowly through gravel and the car doors slamming, and then murmurings. I don't need to see her. Everything will be all right. Craig will be able to go back to work. Mom has returned to help me with the intimate details of recovery while the doctors figure out what the hell is happening to me. I fall asleep listening to her put her bag down near my bed. And then I hear the water running in the kitchen sink. Mom is back. Thank god.

SIXTY-TWO

Turning Corners

"Turning a corner" is a phrase I think about a lot. How will I know when I've turned a corner? Will I turn a corner at all? I mean, of course I will, but still, when? I weigh the options of giving up (although what would that even look like?) versus fighting on. There are only those two options really, to take care of myself and do what the doctors tell me to do, or to give up.

I'm aware that there is a limited amount of all this that I'm in charge of. There are certain things pertaining to my body that I can control. For instance, I can floss and keep my gums healthy. I can support my body. I sleep and dream and stretch. I take little ten-step walks. I drink my water and take my vitamins. I think positive thoughts and listen to cello adagios. I can slow down my heart rate by breathing deeply. But where exactly is the line between what I can and can't affect? Can I heal the sutured incision inside of me? It doesn't feel like I can, but if I can control what I think, if I can control my cortisol levels, say, through meditation, maybe I can control how well that incision heals. I try to make the environment as conducive to healing as humanly possible. I don't blame myself for starting to bleed, though. I can't control that. I would if I could.

From here inside this sick body, I know that I am sick. There is nothing fuzzy or unclear about it. I don't have to check and see if my glands are swollen or if I have a fever the way my parents did when I was little to see if I could go to school. Nope. I am not well. I am, in fact, pretty unwell. There is no mistaking this for wellness.

And I suppose I will know too when I've turned a corner. Like, if you're not sure whether or not you've turned the corner, you probably haven't.

SIXTY-THREE

Percocet

In the middle of the night my eyes pop open. There *is* a third option.

I keep the unused Percocet tablets in my bathroom cabinet. They are my safety net, should I ever end up like my father, needing to be hoisted out of bed by a Hoyer lift and plunked, blind and confused, into a wheelchair to stare at the wall. He didn't want his life to end like that, and I imagine that I will not want it either. I like being alive and all, but even now I'm not ferocious about being alive at any cost. I don't want to live as long as possible, the way some people do.

Craig instructs me, "If I'm even an eyelash on a pillow, keep me alive." Fine for him but not for me.

I asked a doctor friend in an email how many Percocet it would take to kill someone. He responded, "Well, the Tylenol in them could kill you if you took twenty at a time. The oxycodone in it could kill you at about that level, assuming you were not addicted and

therefore tolerant to its sedating and respiratory block-
ing effect. The epidemic of opioid overdoses that the US
is now watching is due to addicts injecting unknown
quantities of unknown opiates. The ingredient listings
on a baggy of heroin are not up to FDA standards."

I just went down and counted. I have twenty-nine
Percocet left. Just in case. I'm covered if it ever, ever
comes to Option Three.

SIXTY-FOUR

"Despairing"

I am a writer, and an archivist by nature. I have all the letters I wrote home from Camp Trywoodie in the seventies. I have a letter that Mister Rogers wrote me in 1981. I am a pack rat when it comes to paper, so when Mom cleans out boxes from her attic, I tend to be the recipient of anything that she feels is important enough to save.

One such packet is an envelope of papers that had belonged to her mother. Grandma Hastings didn't keep a diary, but when she moved to our house in Croton, she was writing on the back of that little Norcross calendar I'd find forty years later. She got it from the drugstore maybe. It has a colorful drawing of a kitten for January, a pink-haired cupid inside a heart for February, a leprechaun and his pot of gold for March. You get the idea. It is from 1969. She died in 1970, but no 1970 calendar is extant.

I keep coming back to the calendar. She has circled dates and written in doctor appointments in tiny handwriting, crammed neatly into the margins of the four-inch-wide calendar pages. She notes *bed* on March eighth, which is when, I assume, her hospital bed was delivered. She marks on the twenty-seventh, *began med.* On April twenty-eighth she's written, *Began Hormones.*

When I turn the pages over, though, she had written more, like a prisoner who has filled up every inch of the slivers of paper they could find. Here she writes *April 3—Dinner with family. Sat at table—exhausted—but no pain increase.* On the back of the calendar's cover, she is keeping track of the dates of what she refers to as her medical crisis.

> *Came to Anne's*   *Jan*
> *Went to Hospital*   *Jan 23*
> *Corset too painful*   *Feb 8*
> *Crisis of pain*   *Feb 10*
> *Back growing more painful—movement more difficult—cannot sustain any light activity like writing—greatly discouraged*   *Feb—20–28*

On the back of January 1969, she wrote and underlined: *weeks of black despair*, and *despairing*. I check with my mother. No, Grandma Hastings never complained, never mentioned sorrow or worries or pain of any kind. She got up every morning, made her Wheatena with three prunes cooked in it, stirred it with a wooden spoon, cleaned the copper-bottomed pot she used. She drove herself to doctor appointments. She didn't want to cause any bother. That's what I think.

Mom has regrets over this. She was so busy with her own four kids running around. We all needed so much, as little children do, and Mom was keenly aware that she didn't have time during those years for her mother, even though she was living with us. They never got to sit quietly and catch up, or surely Mom would have known of her own mother's suffering.

I barely grasped that she was my mother's mother. I just wanted to be near Grandma Hastings, to sleep in her room, to sit with her and eat my grilled cheese sandwiches while watching Julia Child on Grandma's little black-and-white television.

Now as I lie in my daybed staring at the ceiling, I think about her "weeks of black despair." She's been dead for decades, a lifetime now, but I'm still getting to know Grandma Hastings. I think about her many troubles, about her own mother's early death so that she had to be raised by her grandparents, about her fiancé Horton's suicide, and her subsequent decades of spinsterhood until she met my grandfather at forty. I think about her two miscarriages and the baby who only lived a week and is buried now beside my alcoholic grandfather up in Constable, New York.

When I was going through my own miscarriages, I wanted to keep trying, in part for Grandma. She wouldn't have given up, and when I finally did give up, it felt like a rebuke of her determination. I've always felt that I let Grandma Hastings down (in particular) by not having kids because it is the end of not just my own story but of her hard-fought story as well, and of her mother's, and her mother's.

Legacy is such an amorphous concept. Why should I care that her stories die with me? Why should I care whether or not my stories live on? Who cares? It is such narcissism to think our stories matter in the grand scheme of things, but it feels like some kind of biological imperative. The fact that my grandmother's hair reached below her waist is important to me, that she survived yellow fever as a child, that her fiancé killed himself because he had syphilis, that she lay in her bed at night, at the end of her life, "despairing." These stories matter. Don't they? My hope is that writing them down here will cast her line into the future, will be my attempt at securing her story, and possibly mine as well.

Still, "black despair." She was my best friend that year, and she was suffering, and nobody knew.

SIXTY-FIVE

Scalpel vs Bullet

When I expressed surprise over how stunned my body felt after surgery, how long it was taking me to even want to walk around, one of my besties said, "Your body doesn't know the difference between a scalpel and a bullet."

Jesus. But she's right. If I had been stabbed, I guess I wouldn't have felt like I had to hurry up and get better, wouldn't have felt like I should immediately begin weaning myself off the ibuprofen and run a marathon or something. Yes, surgery can be as physically traumatic as being shot.

I see now I'm part of a cultural phenomenon in which we don't feel like we can admit that we're ever sick, ever tired, ever injured. We don't know how to rest. It's all "Hurry up and get back to work." It's all, "Stop complaining."

But I sat and watched the little bruise from the IV on the back my hand. It was the only injury that I could see from the surgery, and that bruise took almost two weeks to fade from black to purple to yellow to gone, and that was from one stupid little needle prick, not being cut open and having internal organs manhandled and snipped out. Healing takes time. Living takes time. I like resting now. I have respect for people who know how to rest.

SIXTY-SIX

The Depths

I don't know how long it's been since surgery, several weeks? But one night around 3:00 a.m. I bleed an alarming amount. I sleep in twenty-minute increments, jolting awake when it seems like I'm about to ruin the mattress . . . AGAIN.

I see the doctors every single day to determine if I need to be transfused. I am getting weaker. I am on bed-rest, but I feel like maybe I should be in the hospital. I don't know.

One day I arrive at the doctor's office to see Dr. G but when I get there, I learn he's had to go into emergency surgery. I have to sit for two hours in air-conditioning. Craig leaves me there. He has to go to work. I rest with my hands on the cane, my head resting on the back of my hands, and become very still, powering down. I tell myself to just let the cold air and time move past me. Be a rock in a stream.

When it's all over, a friend has to pick me up and take me home, where I collapse. *Collapse* is too energetic a word. I crumble? I evanesce? Somehow I get inside the house from the car and I ease into the daybed, I don't remember how, and the covers come up around me and then I am waking up, and there is Zonker, and there is my mom with a pill, and I feel blood so my body gets up and into the bathroom, doubles over, face pressed to knees. When I am gone in the bathroom, Mom straightens up the pad we have over the bed, retucks my sheets, and readies a tiny bowl of applesauce (all I want to eat now, or celery broth, one or the other) and whatever meds I am scheduled to take.

How would I get through this alone? I don't know.

When I get into bed, I lie on my side, a pillow pressed to my stomach to hold everything in place. With my other arm, I hug myself and say something encouraging. I am inside my body, but we are two different things— my awareness is one thing, my body is something else. Me and my body seem to be slipping further and further away from one another. I praise my body for trying to heal, for showing grace under pressure, while being aware that it is me encouraging myself.

Because the doctor keeps asking me about the color and consistency of the blood, I bring one of the soaked pads to him so that he can decide what color the blood is and what it means. I tell him to smell the pad. No kidding. We're detectives and sort of desperate. If we don't figure this out, if the bleeding doesn't stop and the bedrest doesn't help, the next step is being readmitted. The blood on the pad smells to me like the blood from hamburger meat sloshing in the bottom of those shrink-wrapped, Styrofoam containers in the supermarket. That seems like it could be useful diagnostic information. It doesn't smell like new blood, in other words. The doctor is not disgusted that I brought the bloody pad in, or at least he doesn't seem grossed out. He calls the other two doctors in, in fact, and they gather around the pad and look at it and smell it. This is what we've come to. Sheesh. No one has answers, and we sit there saying how much we hope my body can fix this, whatever it is, because the thought of cutting me open again to find out where I am bleeding sounds like murder.

And so the days advance.

SIXTY-SEVEN

The Dissection

Grandma Hastings studied biology at Sophie Newcomb, and was a lab technician for a while, before becoming a biology teacher.

So it was not out of character when she decided to dissect a frog on the breakfast room table for us kids in 1969. She was eighty by then, and it had been a good sixty years since she had studied biology in New Orleans. It was maybe fifty years since she'd worked in a lab, and maybe forty since she'd taught schoolchildren to delineate between different kinds of clouds, and how the planets orbit around the sun.

She asked my brothers to catch her a frog, which she put in a shoebox, which she slid into the freezer. She wanted to show us how frogs went dormant in winter, and this I do remember (although most of the rest I think I only know because this story has been retold to me so many times over the years). She said that in winter, frogs could dig down in the mud by our pond and had something like antifreeze in their veins so that they wouldn't freeze solid, but would instead go into a kind of torpor, something like the way bears hibernate.

Her operating theater was a piece of cardboard and T-shaped sewing pins on the breakfast room table. She had a little jar of chloroform and a piece of cotton, and she had a scalpel (I'm pretty sure that I don't actually remember this part), and when she took the frozen frog out of the shoebox, she cut him down his white abdomen and very neatly pinned back his skin to reveal his frozen but still slowly beating heart along with his inflating and deflating lungs. We must have crowded around that table, four kids ranging in age from five to fourteen, craning our necks to see what she was quietly, authoritatively pointing at. The cruelty of it, the fact that it was vivisection, never occurred to me until now.

For most of my life I thought that Grandma Hastings stitched that frog up, nursed him back to health, and set him free. I feel like I saw him hopping away in our backyard toward Teatown Lake, but who can explain memory and its vagaries. I was in my forties when my mother disabused me of that fairy tale. "How on earth would she be able to sew him up and nurse him back to health?" She choked, she was laughing so hard. "My mother nursed a frog back from open-heart surgery? Not likely."

I don't think anyone would have lied to me about it. We had plenty of evidence of the cold-hearted natural world. For a year, we'd cared for an orphaned deer who was then killed by neighborhood dogs. My mother took care of a neighbor's pet boa constrictor that had a fungal infection and she had to dip its head in hydrogen peroxide twice a day (she's a badass). The chickens were regularly picked off by fox and skunks and raccoons (and probably neighborhood dogs—there were no leash laws in Westchester County in the 1970s). I'd once held a dying robin in my hands that I'd found on the ground, already close to death under the blue spruce tree. I'd cupped it in my hands, petting its rising chest softly with my pointer finger as it slowly stopped breathing. I watched the life leak out, its eyes going gray, its spirit effervescing. So I think I could have handled the frog's post-dissection death, and I was surprised decades later to learn the truth, surprised that I had invented a happy ending for the frog. What a little romantic I'd been.

But I remember being with my oldest brother. He was driving us to the North Shore on Oahu, where he's lived most of his adult life. I brought up Grandma Hastings' famous frog dissection, and without skipping a beat, Bradley says, "and she sutured him up and he hopped away!" Is he right? Is Mom? Brad was fourteen when she dissected that frog. He's the one who caught it for her, for god's sake. He's got the eye of a naturalist too, and so now I don't know which version is true, but I want to believe his. I want Grandma to have helped the frog live after open-heart surgery.

SIXTY-EIGHT

My Corner

Sassafras trees grow from 9–35 m (30–115 ft) tall with many slender sympodial branches, and smooth, orange-brown bark or yellow bark. All parts of the plants are fragrant. The species are unusual in having three distinct leaf patterns on the same plant: unlobed oval, bilobed (mitten-shaped), and trilobed (three-pronged) . . .

—Wikipedia

One morning I look around and realize that I've turned a corner. The blood is slowing. I sit up and watch the morning weather report with Mom and Craig and don't go back to sleep until around 8:00 p.m.

The next day Mom and I are back on the lawn with our chairs and our books. I want to walk to the mailbox, so Mom and I walk down together. For the first time in a while I see our little sassafras tree, its leaves still clinging. I remember being six or seven years old, and

Warren teaching us how to identify the three different leaves that a sassafras has all those years ago on the Wildflower Island in Teatown Lake. "One leaf looks like a mitten." Oh, it's nice to be outside in the fall, and I feel so good that I even carry the mail up in one hand, my other holding the walking stick.

I feel a general surge of excitement. I want to go upstairs, but Craig tells me to wait. I start thinking about walking back to the monks' driveway, just a few drive-ways down the road, but that seems too far, so I wait.

And Zonker knows too, because he jumps up on the daybed but no longer stays by my feet. He comes up by my face now, and his sister Crinkle comes up too. The three of us cram into the daybed together, and I move on apace.

Mom will leave soon, and I know this time it will be for keeps. Am I ready for her to go? The people we love move away from us. I might be ready.

The blood is there still, but slowing, sometimes almost to nothing, like that dried-up stream I saw near the abbey on the hill. I still wear a pad. It's been months and months and months now that I've worn pads, but I have down-graded to the thinner ones—not the thinnest but thinner. There is no underwear left to ruin. I start thinking about buying new underwear. That's a good sign.

AN OLD FRIEND of my father is very sick. She posts on Facebook asking for prayers. When I post about having turned a corner, she is excited to know that there may be a corner for her to turn too. A few months later, she finds that her medical journey does not have a corner to turn. By the following May she is dead. Her death is a shock, and reminds me of how frail we are, and of how much I want to get better.

SIXTY-NINE

Women of a Certain Age

People keep asking me if I'm sad. They say, "How are you feeling?" and tilt their heads and get these big sad eyes. I get it. People want me to mourn the end of my reproductive possibilities. They expect me to be devastated, to feel like less of a woman. There's plenty for me to feel bad about, I guess, but at the moment I'm not upset, and specifically not upset about fertility issues. I just want to be well. I can't be devastated on command.

I search inside myself to see if I feel different about my body without a uterus. I was a "childless woman" before the surgery, but this is, of course, a final shutting of that door. I know I am supposed to be reassessing, but search though I do, I can't feel what I think I'm supposed to be feeling, that I am less in some way, diminished. It's like trying to cry at a sad movie. I can't force it, and really, I'm kind of liking my body, which is finally healing. I'm amazed at what a body can accomplish.

WOMEN HAD WARNED me that I would become invisible at fifty, that men would not want me or even see me, that the world would treat me as irrelevant. I'm already in my fifties and wonder: *Can this be true?*

Well, it's true that my legs are never as smooth as they once were, no matter how I shave or moisturize, and men do not catcall, do not shout things out at me in the street anymore. But smooth legs and catcalls are a whole different kind of invisibility, right? I'm relieved to have those days of being just a flower that lures bees over and done with.

There may no longer be lines of giddy men wanting to sleep with me, but I feel pretty alive. I don't feel invisible. I feel sort of smoking hot, in my own middle-aged way. I know I'm not technically fertile or anything, but shit, I feel fertile, feel overflowing with ideas and love for the world. I stick a sprig of mint in a glass by the sink and two days later, there are roots reaching an inch into the water. I do the same with a branch of basil from the grocery store. Same thing. Having kids is one kind of fertility, but it's dawning on me that there's more than one way to be fruitful.

When I went to New Orleans a few Augusts ago, there was a drunk splayed out on the cobblestones of the French Quarter at 6:00 a.m. It was ninety-seven degrees already, and this guy on the ground was radiating the night's worth of alcohol (or whatever) he'd ingested. His feet were cracked and caked with dirt, and he looked up at me through his red-rimmed, crusted eyes and said, "Mornin' beautiful." Just like that. "Mornin' beautiful," in his slurred bass voice. I knew he couldn't see me, that his eyes couldn't even focus in the morning light. I knew he was just a drunk guy almost passed out from whatever sledgehammer he'd used to shut down the world. But I didn't care. It was nice. Yes. I thought it was nice.

It felt like his eyes were remembering something from a long time ago, and for some reason, silly as it seems, I felt seen by him. And what's more, I saw *him*. It was like he had an angel or a ghost or something smiling through him right at me. And he could see how beautiful I was. I loved this man.

Even now, I delight in every door held open for me. How marvelous it all is—the drunks and the doormen. My husband sees me. I see myself. I may not feel well, but I don't feel invisible, and even with an unwell body, I swear that I have never felt more trembling on the edge of the sky, never felt more essentially seen and alive.

I refuse what some women warn me of—that no longer being sexually alluring makes me dust or something. I am too busy beaming and being dazzled while the world shimmers around me like a giant ball of tangled yarn.

SEVENTY

Egg Sacs

There are four life stages in an insect's life cycle. If it completes all four stages of a life cycle the individual species is said to complete a metamorphosis stage. However, not every species undergoes a complete metamorphosis. There are some that [have] only three life stages. [The] praying mantis is one of them. Furthermore, the mantis doesn't only undergo an incomplete metamorphosis—the young and adult mantises look almost entirely the same.

—Praying-mantis.org

I feel better enough to google *praying mantis*. It's the end of October now and with the chilly air, it's nice to be curious about something, and to think of someone other than myself, even if that someone else is a praying mantis.

I read to Mom from the internet, "The adult [mantids] can't survive freezing temperatures." Uh-oh. "Looks like they only live for one year, and it looks like by this time of year only females are still around. I guess Claude is a female."

"He's still Claude to me," she says, and I agree. He will always be Claude to me.

"It says here he's going to lay his egg sac soon." I paraphrase from the internet: "Looks like in cold-weather climates, they ensure the survival of their species by laying hundreds of eggs that are essentially glued together in an egg case called an ootheca."

We're both quiet for a few minutes, sipping our coffee and taking in the information.

"Well, it seems like after that they die pretty soon," I say.

"Maybe we should put him outside," Mom says. "We don't want him to lay his eggs in here." I like that she's still calling him "him." "When those eggs hatch in the spring, they should be outside or they'll die." She's right.

We get up and go stand by where Claude is perched in the Christmas cactus. He's hanging upside down, horrifying and paralyzed as ever, and enormous. I can see that he's plump like he's full of hundreds of eggs.

Mom says, "Get the door," so I open the door to the outside. She uses her fingers like little pincers and picks

Claude up from behind. He is big and writhing and clearly hates being touched. Maybe he thinks Mom is a crow about to eat him. "Oh!" she says, "he's grabbing at me with his hind legs." Yuk. She reaches outside the sunroom door and places him on the azalea bush just there across from the now gone-to-seed garden.

"I'm impressed," I tell her, not sure that I'd want to have been the one to put him outside. Mom should have been an ambulance driver in a war, or one of those guys who disables bombs. She looks sweet, but she can dip a boa's head in hydrogen peroxide. She shouldn't be underestimated.

"Oh look!" she says, and we both lean toward where Claude is clinging to a narrow branch of the azalea bush. It's not even two minutes since Mom put him outside, and he's already begun laying his egg sac under a clump of leaves, conveniently for us at eye level. He's moving kind of slowly, pulling these foamy eggs out of his distended abdomen with his back legs. We watch, then go inside, then go back outside to watch some more. It takes him hours to get all of the foamy eggs out and into a clump, suspended from the underside of an azalea leaf.

I read to Mom from the internet: "This says farmers

buy egg sacs because mantids are good for farmland and gardens. They help get rid of pests."

Claude will die soon. That's what happens once they lay their eggs, but I will look for Claude's babies come the spring. They can help me in next year's garden.

SEVENTY-ONE

Mom Leaves for Real

And all of a sudden, just like that, the worst is over. My hemoglobin rises from 6-point-something to 8, and then to a little over 8, and then almost to 9. That change raises my energy and optimism. I am less fearful with all of this hemoglobin rushing around in my blood.

There is a moment when Mom and I both know she can go home. Maybe it's after walking up and down the driveway, hardly leaning on my stick at all. Maybe it's when I have an appetite again. (I go to the freezer and eat the entire pint of sea-salt caramel ice cream that my friend Kathy brought when I was sick. I eat it standing up in the middle of the kitchen.) I keep wondering how I would have made it without Mom.

It seems especially lucky to have had this time with her as a grown woman. All of her healing ways, and her mother's too I suppose, are imprinted on my brain now, for when I need them later, for when, one day (ugh!), I'm unwell again and Mom can no longer be with me.

But it is time. She and Craig are getting ever-so-slightly on each other's nerves, the way troops do when the battle's done. Mom has taken over because I needed her to, and now is the right moment for Craig and me to regain our private equilibrium. And she has a lot to get back to as well. She's let her whole life slide to take care of me. There are friends for her to see and her own bills to pay and thank-you cards to write. She packs up and leaves now for the second time, my sister's boyfriend again driving an hour each way to get her and take her home.

I stand in the driveway and say, "Goodbye." Mom sticks her head out of the car window. "What?" she says. I laugh and shout, "GOODBYE."

She says goodbye and waves, and I wave back, but neither of us cries this time. No. I go inside and make tea. I imagine that when she gets home, she'll immediately start going through her mail before she even takes off her coat.

MY FRIEND SHAY says that happiness is an act of courage. Her dad told her that, and maybe someone famous said it before him. I don't know, but in high school, Shay told me.

I'm repeating here what my friend Shay's father told Shay, and what my friend Shay then told me . . . "Happiness is an act of courage." I say it because I find it to be true.

Shay also told me, "The people we love move away from us," a fact that leads to so much suffering. Some move away by dying, and others to follow their dreams elsewhere. Others move away because their love has vanished. As Dickens wrote in *Great Expectations* (a book that Dad and I read to one another many years ago): "Life is made of ever so many partings welded together." Mom has gone. I am, at last, well.

Part Six

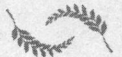

No One but Us

SEVENTY-TWO

Almost Upstairs

I start organizing the sheaves of paper from doctors and insurance companies. And then I nap, but only for two hours this time. I walk down to the mailbox twice that first day after Mom leaves. The next day I walk to the monks' mailbox. The day after that I walk there twice. And so on.

On Saturday, Craig takes me to the supermarket to go shopping for the first time in a couple of months. The walk from the parking lot to the carts is so enormously long I don't know how I failed to notice it before. I push my cart through the riotous vegetables and fruit. Too much. Too much. I put a little container of cut-up pineapple in my cart, and then I freeze. I don't want to move farther away from the door, so I just stand there next to the nuts and popcorn, still in aisle one, and wait for Craig to come find me. When we get home it's a three-plus-hour nap this time.

Craig sleeps on the couch in the living room. I've said I can come upstairs. I've said that he can sleep up there even if I can't quite, but he thinks I need one more night downstairs and he wants to keep me company. "There's no rush," he says. "You're getting better. There's no rush. No rush." His lack of pressure draws me to him.

I lie in the daybed, the cats and five pillows crushed around me, and I can hear Craig breathing on the couch nearby. I begin to look forward again to sharing a bed with him. I am not afraid of him turning over and me being caught by a flung elbow. I am no longer afraid of his hugging me too hard. It all sounds lovely, being bunched up in bed with him next to me again.

Longing unfolds in me as my body heals. There is a lot to get better for. We are ever so slowly getting back into the rhythm of just the two of us in the house. He is singing in the shower again. I can call upstairs to him and he can shout back down. We leave the mail on the table. Craig can drink right out of the milk carton. We don't do these things when we have visitors.

SEVENTY-THREE

No Rush, No Rush

Craig drives me to my final checkup and waits in the waiting room. Dr. S tells me that I'm good to go. He is so relieved that my body has won this campaign. "Can I drive now?" I ask him. Yes. "Can I lift things?" Yes, but nothing over five pounds for a while. "Can I have sex?" I ask. He pauses.

"The thing with sex is," he says, looking over the top of his little wire-rimmed glasses at me, "if you want to, go ahead. If you don't, don't." He shrugs. I love him. I really do. I don't know then that I'll never see this man again. Another farewell.

The next day I get into my car and drive all alone to the grocery store. It is so overwhelming to drive in actual traffic that, after I park the car and turn off the engine, I sit for a bit in the parking lot, turn the car back on, and drive home. That was enough. No rush. No rush.

The next day I try again. I park. I get a cart. I walk in and get an apple. I have a list but I start to feel worried. I'm all alone and the walk back to the car, the drive back home, the walk from the car to the house all seem perilous and kaleidoscopic. So I only get three of the seven items on the list: an apple, half-and-half for my coffee, more organic unsweetened applesauce. That's enough. I lean against something at checkout. It seems to take forever and I am overcome by fatigue, but I now know how to become still, how to hold on to my energy. I hold on. I don't make a lot of eye contact. I get my money out ahead of time.

I get through checkout and walk slowly to my car. There is a small uphill stretch in the parking lot that I never noticed before. It is a lot more work to walk uphill. I rest in the car for a few minutes. Then I drive the three miles home. Will I ever again be impatient with slow-moving people?

And in bite-sized increments I get through the first weeks of actual recovery, hitting little milestones along the way. I move back into our bed upstairs with the whole gang: Craig and Zonker and Crinkle and me. Craig puts on old episodes of *The Mary Tyler Moore Show* to help me fall asleep at night. I feel mostly OK, with who knows how much healing still to do, but back and alive and happy. The worst is over, and whatever *this* stage is, I'll get through this too.

SEVENTY-FOUR

To the Abbey

My favorite goal on my giant To Do list is to walk closer to the abbey. I have gotten a few feet up the big first hill, but I haven't felt ready for the big hill. Then, one day, I make it up the big hill, ever so slowly, my breath coming in big heaves. My hemoglobin levels are still around 8. While they're higher than they were, they aren't where they should be yet, and I'm exhausted. (Below 12 grams of hemoglobin per milliliter is apparently considered low, but I learn later that doctors don't transfuse a patient until the hemoglobin is below 6, or if the patient has a heart condition and won't tolerate anemia. This is why I was getting finger pricks every time I went to the doctor, because at a hemoglobin level of under 7, I was borderline transfusable.)

So I MAKE it to the top of the hill and feel as though I've summited Mount Everest. I look around, my walking stick in my hand. I want to plant a flag. Instead, I turn and walk back down the big hill and up the road to my driveway, and up my driveway, and into my house and straight to bed.

A few days later I push myself. As I trudge up the hill, my lungs burning, I count my steps, and remember what Dad taught me as a kid. We'd go on bicycle rides through mountainous Westchester County (no helmets back in the 1970s), and on the killer inclines he'd say, "Don't look at the top of the hill. It's too daunting. Just look down at your feet and pedal." Dad has been dead for several years now, but still he's with me. I look down at my feet and count my steps. I twirl Grandma Hastings' wedding ring on my finger.

I pause then and decide I can keep going all the way to the abbey itself. It has been maybe two months since I've been all the way to the abbey. The leaves are mostly gone from the trees. I come to the fork and take the gravel road toward the abbey. The little pile of rocks I made is still there. There is no hat hanging from a branch, but the rusted exhaust pipe is where I last saw it.

At the abbey I see no people at first, but the work they've done on the bell tower is astonishing. It looks almost finished. A man comes out, not a monk, a man in civilian clothes. I've seen him before. I think he lives in the trailer just to the side. "It looks so good," I tell him, leaving it at that. He gives me a tour.

"There are other monks coming soon for their annual meeting," he tells me, "so we wanted to get this done for them to see." He's proud of his work and points out the way he has finished the concrete walls with a nice, rounded hump at the top. He shows me the planters he has built into the walls. "We can plant something pretty there in the spring," he says. I feel metaphors everywhere.

"What about the bell?" I ask. It's a bell tower, after all, that they've been building all this time.

"Someone's donating one, that's what they told me. So the bell tower's done, but no bell yet." *Metaphors metaphors metaphors.* A bell tower with no bell. Planters ready now for flowers come spring. Me too, I want to say. Me too.

I've made it to the abbey and that is far enough. I shouldn't stay and talk too long, as the journey back seems a challenging one, so I say goodbye. When I am at the top of the big hill, heading back toward home, there is a tremendous uprush of wind. I let the leaves swirl around me, the wind so strong that my hair is swept up in the air.

It feels like the forest is saying, "welcome" and "welcome" and "welcome." It is pleasant to feel invited into the future.

SEVENTY-FIVE

Reminders

My mother found a photograph of Horton, her mother's first love, when Mom was just a little girl. She asked her mother about it, and to Mom's dismay, Grandma started to cry, so Mom never mentioned it again. But when Grandma died, my mother found that old photograph of Horton and burned it in the fireplace while Grandma was being cremated. Two curls of smoke.

Years later I found Horton's obituary, and online I found a photograph of his grave, also in New Orleans but at Lafayette Cemetery No. 1. I have thought many times of having him reinterred with Grandma in Metairie, but who am I to disturb the dead?

Why do these things matter to me? Why am I putting them here? She was a real person is all, and I have no children to tell these stories to. I put her stories here because I am passing them on, keeping her alive. She was loved by someone once, not the man she would eventually marry, not the alcoholic philanderer. She was in love with Horton, and would love him for a life-time, despite his suicide. Just as I drag her with me, she dragged Horton with her, so now I carry them both.

SEVENTY-SIX

An Adventure

Not long after my surgery, I get an email from an artist-friend in Holland inviting me to housesit for them while they're in Iceland. I can't quite believe it, it's so out of the blue. I met her and her family in Ireland two Christmases before, at an artists' residency on the cliffs of County Kerry. We'd spent Christmas and New Year's Eve together, had gone into the little town of Cahirsiveen and sipped hot chocolate on a cold rainy December day at a pub. We had become friends.

Holland. I'd never been to Holland. I'd never really thought about going to Holland. But it sounded like magic. When Craig came down, I read him the email. I asked him what he thought.

"Well, you'll be homesick, but you'll get a lot of writing done. And you could use an adventure."

I thought about it. I didn't even know what language they spoke in Holland, or where it was on the map. I didn't know if I'd be well enough to travel, if I'd be strong enough to carry my suitcase around. I had no money (except for savings), no job lined up for the fall.

"Yes," I wrote back that day. "If you really mean it, the answer is YES!" I will spend the month of March there.

Saying yes to this feels like a test of whether or not I deserve to be well. I feel an enormous urge to say yes to things, to assert my wellness. If I am going to be alive, I want to have adventures. So I say yes.

Yes. Yes. Yes.

If illness is about living the narrowed focus of a single bed, then for me, wellness will be about opening my focus wide, wider than the house, the yard, the state, wider than the country even.

SEVENTY-SEVEN

Mom's Answer

Much later, Mom sends me the following email. She wrote it exactly as follows.

From: Anne Moss
To: West Moss
Subject: old age minus kids

It's an interesting question that West posed: Supposing I had no offspring how would I choose to fill my time?

Having one abiding interest is helpful. I worked on stained glass from the 1970s to around 2008. That got me way past retirement age.

An instance many years before that might give a clue to an answer. I spent a year off and on being a tourist and student in the city. I took many bus tours, signed up for a class in fiction writing at the New School, and went to regular lectures at the

MET, based only on what they were offering, not on any particular interest of mine. That's a good way to expand one's horizons.

I am not a philanthropist in any meaning of the word. I don't want to be on the Board of some admired cause, don't want to go to patron dinners. I am not a joiner. Those parameters leave one with friends and acquaintances only. That's not enough to fill one's time nor is it rewarding in opening up new worlds because we tend to stick with "birds of a feather" which supply a needed comfort level and certain companionship. So, what I think I would find myself doing is the following:

I'd make my world smaller, sell the house and probably move to the city where a wealth of possibilities exist. The 92nd Street Y, whose catalogue of events I just received (the size of a small phone book) offers endless lectures and musical events. All the museums have lectures. There are some college classes that can be audited. I'd love that. Libraries offer exhibits and lectures. Some of these adventures cost money, some are free but one can work within one's budget. I think it's also wise to have schedules in place. This means signing up for something that meets every Wednesday at noon for example. It's easy to be lazy and say, it's hot I don't feel like going out. With appointments in place it's not good to weasel out.

The above takes care of intellectual fodder but there needs to be time for play. That's where one gets back to friends. Go to movies, and occasional documentaries with someone so there can be a discussion later. Have a meal in the park or at a restaurant with a friend and maybe that friend has another friend to bring. Go to a concert or musical event with someone.

All those ideas are dependent on one's well being. What happens when one can function in only a limited way and we've reached the stage where all we're trying to do is kill time until we die? When most abilities have failed then one is lucky to be able to read, write letters and watch TV, never once moving out of one location. One of the saddest revelations I had in viewing the inmates at SkyView [the nursing home where my father died] was that only one among the many, many I saw, carried and read a book. Why was no one else reading? Why was no one ever watching the continuously running TVs? They weren't all totally out of it. My guess is that those who had their wits to some degree had reached that stage where they were just filling time before kicking off and everything was too much trouble, except eating.

p.s. The truth of the matter is that YOU would and will, in the future, do just fine under your own personal tutelage. You've never lacked for innovative ideas and you have an innate sense for the importance of staying in touch with people.

Part Seven

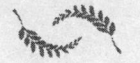

Holland and Beyond

SEVENTY-EIGHT

Eindhoven

A few months after surgery, I leave for Holland. It is, perhaps, a crazy thing to do. But the bleeding has stopped for real, and I can lift my own suitcase when necessary. I have an up-to-date passport. Nothing specific is holding me back. I feel uncertain, but not enough to keep me here.

My palpable longing for adventure has been growing after being cooped up for so long. This is another stage of the healing process—feeling ready to go out into the wider world. I want to go beyond the borders of New York and New Jersey. I feel a longing to escape the boundaries of my body and of our house.

And so Craig drives me over the Whitestone Bridge to JFK Airport (you know a man loves you when he drives you to JFK Airport), and off I go.

The trip to Holland is complicated and full of ups and downs. I learn that a friend from college lives very close to where I'll be staying, and she, Buffi, meets me at the airport with a giant bunch of tulips and anemones. She drives me past windmills and right to the door of my home-away-from-home in the suburbs of Eindhoven. Buffi is like sunshine for an anxious traveler.

My hosts, who will only overlap with me for twenty-four hours before leaving for their own adventure in Iceland, greet me with what I come to understand is a Dutch gift of quiet but overflowing hospitality. For breakfast Mels makes me cappuccino and toast with butter and chocolate sprinkles on it. Why is this not a thing in the US? Marielle takes me for a bike ride into Eindhoven proper to show me the train station, and where I can safely leave my bicycle in the enormous, free underground bicycle parking lot. We sit over coffee in a store talking and talking and talking, trying to catch up in the little time we have together, sharing all of the highlights and sorrows of one another's lives that are inappropriate to share electronically. I want to hold her hands every second that we're together. Right after I think this, she takes my hand and we don't let go.

But they have to leave early the next morning, and I feel both relief to be on my own and a rising panic. There is a lot to remember: their address, how to get to the train, how the dishwasher works, and the shower, and the front door lock. I am far away from home, all on my own. It is all up to me. If I get locked out, what will I do? Who will I call?

I have to stay alert because a friend of mine is flying from Paris and will meet me the next day in Amsterdam where I've booked a room in a B&B for the night. First my hosts leave and then I leave the house a few hours later, with instructions scribbled on a piece of paper. My backpack is full of phone numbers, addresses, and maps, and I walk the mile or so to the train station in a cold mist, and the train isn't where it is supposed to be. Thus begins one of my hardest days. I find the train, eventually, my heart racing now, and remain on alert the entire hour or so trip into Amsterdam. I am so alert every second of that day that I am already exhausted by the time I arrive in Amsterdam, where I get a text from my friend who is supposed to be meeting me there. Instead, she says I should take the metro to where she is. I hadn't expected that, so I scramble around and ask five different people the same question for directions, and I find my way to the metro, buy a ticket, and get to the right stop.

I should mention that I've purchased my first smart phone ever for this trip, and I'm not confident about how it works. In fact, I inadvertently use up all of my data in one day, and learn only then that I have to turn off the international roaming, but from there on out, I'm barely using the phone for backup because I don't want to have to pay for extra international data. I know that I can't make any phone calls without paying an exorbitant fee, so I'm using it not for GPS or the internet, but just for texting. This all adds to my strangled feeling of being alone and far away from help, cut off.

It is raining when I come up aboveground from the metro, and it's a cold rain. The wind is blowing and I'm wearing all the wrong clothes. My coat is soaked through in three seconds, and my baseball cap (because I hadn't brought an umbrella) is dripping from the brim almost immediately. My friend, Whitney, meets me there and we walk and chatter and get completely lost together, me carrying all my stuff with me. It is perhaps 10:00 a.m. and I am already freezing and uncertain, feeling a very tentative and iffy tether back to my home-away-from-home in Eindhoven, and an even less palpable tether back to my own country, house, and husband.

Whitney and I walk to my bed-and-breakfast, which even in daytime is almost impossible to find down some dark alleys off a canal. And it is claustrophobic in there, with tiny steep stairs to climb and cramped quarters inside. But in for a penny, in for a pound. I leave my bag in my room and we go out for an Indian dinner in Amsterdam.

It is after we finish eating that the night reaches its nadir. Whitney goes off to her hotel and I head the few blocks to my B&B, only it isn't there, and now it is dark out, and raining again. I am freezing. In that moment, I realize that I am not 100 percent well after all, and I start to shiver the way I did back when I would let my ibuprofen lapse postsurgery. I get turned around. My hands are shaking. The GPS on my phone isn't working (truth is, I don't know how to use it), and when I stop people on the street who try to be helpful, they can't find the address on their GPS anyway. One guy in a pizza shop sends me in the wrong direction. I am freezing, exhausted, lonely, and I am afraid now too.

Two full hours pass and I don't know where I am, when finally I find the right street. My hands fumble with the keys, and by the time I climb the two steep flights of stairs up to my room, I have what I guess is a panic attack. I can't breathe. I am sweating and crying and know that I cannot sleep in this tiny room. I text Craig, but he rarely has his phone with him and I get no answer. I can't breathe. I briefly think about using my laptop to get some friend to Skype with me, but I can't find the Wi-Fi code in the B&B paperwork, and my panic is continuing to rise. I can hardly stand in the room without shrieking. So I text my sister and she is there! She is there!

I try to convey to her via text what is happening, how I'm feeling. At first she misunderstands and starts to give me advice about GPS software I should use next time I travel, but I text her, "I need you to help me calm down," and bless her peaceful little self, she starts to write out visualizations of me being safe and calm. She's a lifeline, and her communicating with me from so far away calms me just enough so that I can make a plan. I pack up my stuff and in my soaking wet coat I venture back down the dark, steep, coffin-like staircase and head out into the rainy night. Better to sleep on the street in the rain than to be suffocated by the darkness of that little room.

It's late now, well after midnight, and still raining, and there are not many people on the street. I'm lugging my suitcase and my backpack with me, and finally find a woman on the street. My tongue a dry clapper in my mouth, I ask, "Do you speak English?" and then, "How can I get a cab?" She smiles and points over my shoulder, and there, right behind me under a halo-like streetlight is a cab. I get in and burst into tears. The driver gets out and comes to my door. He opens it, and I think he is kicking me out for being hysterical. I briefly consider peacefully resisting him. But no. He stands by my open door with his arms held wide apart. He wants to hug me. I get up and put my head on his shoulder and just sob. He pats my back and says it will be all right. I cry now with relief in the dark drizzle of this Amsterdam night.

In the car he shares his food with me (I am still not sure what we eat . . . it is crunchy and salty), and he takes me to Whitney's hotel. People have warned me that Amsterdam cabbies love to rip tourists off, but I don't care how much he charges me, and of course when we pull up to the hotel the meter reads just fifteen euros, which seems hardly enough for what he's given me. I give him a big tip. In fact I give him all of the money in my pocket, which is twenty-five euros. If I'd had more with me, I would have given it to him. Then he waits outside the hotel, a few feet away, his headlights shining on the hotel's front doors until he sees that I've made it inside.

I've been texting Whitney throughout my ordeal, and she is waiting in the lobby with the concierge. They have a fire going and a cold glass of gin waiting for me. The blessings of the night begin to pile on top of the mess, doing their best to submerge it. The highs and the lows are irreconcilable. Whitney lets me sleep in her bed. Lovely, kind Whitney.

Again I am reminded that the world has avalanches of kindness waiting for me. Later Buffi scolds me. "Next time you get lost, call me and I will come find you wherever you are."

THE NEXT DAY I act calm. I convince myself that I am fine, but I'm still shaken up in a way that won't dissipate for a full week. Back at home I might have taken twenty-four hours to rest and recover from a night like that, but I am in Amsterdam with my friend for just one more day before she goes back to Paris and I return to Eindhoven, so I soldier on. We go to the Van Gogh Museum, where I see his peasants bent over in the fragile light of the fields and his dying sunflowers. I stare at the figures in his *Potato Eaters*, who seem like they're being crushed by the darkness around them. I feel my own panic rising again just thinking about how, when they blow out that single lantern, the darkness will swallow them whole.

Afterward we go to the Anne Frank House just a few streets away, but as we stand in the ever-narrowing space to get to her hidden bedroom, I begin to sweat. There is a black-and-white newsreel playing. The images are of the emaciated, naked cadavers piled outside a concentration camp. They are being pushed into pits by a tractor as though they are sticks of lumber. I feel the grisliest pall start to settle over me, and under it my own panic from the night before is still thrumming like a nest of furious wasps that is being stirred. The walls of this already claustrophobic space feel as though they are leaning in on me, and the sorrow of this young girl, this writer, and the enormity of her personal tragedy and the monstrousness that humanity is capable of all settle down on my shoulders like the walls of a coffin closing in on me. When I consider climbing the stairs into her tiny space, the place where she hid and then was pulled from and taken to the concentration camps, I can't do it, can't willingly lift myself up the last narrow stairs into where she was hidden for twenty-five months.

Whitney and I go instead to a little pub tucked in at the edge of a canal and sit at their long copper bar. We drink beer and order cheese plates, eating and drinking and chatting for hours, my pulse coming back into the neighborhood of normal. We talk and talk and talk, and I am dimly aware that my intense vulnerability here, hidden just below the surface, has somehow made my time with Whitney more important and vivid. She has become a friend for life over these twenty-four hours, having been in the trenches with me thus. And I know that my sister has saved me, just as much as Whitney has, and the cab driver. Why didn't I ask him for his card? I will never see him again, which saddens me. He's someone I'd like to thank.

SEVENTY-NINE

A. L. Snijders

When I get back to Eindhoven, I am coughing, sneezing, and feverish. I go to the grocery store and get what I'm pretty sure is cold medicine. (Most of the people in Holland speak some English, but all the packaging in the stores is in Dutch.) I get cut-up pineapple and tissues and carry it all back to the house, where I lock the door behind me and settle in to just rest and try to calm myself down for a few days.

I am sick and lonely and feel horribly far away from home. I continue to feel a little bit trapped and frantic. I want to go home, but I can't really leave now unless I spend a ton of money and admit defeat. I have to go on, or so it feels. I have three weeks left. I've only just started this trip. There is a six-hour time difference, and Craig and I finally figure out a good time to Skype, and that helps. My longing to climb home through my computer is acute.

After several days of rest and healing, I begin to feel better. My anxiety has dulled, and I feel ready to get my bearings now, to take a trip to the grocery store and learn the names of the streets. Soon I can get to the grocery store and back without writing out the directions. I've figured out how to use the washing machine and how the front door lock works. It's all coming into focus.

I start to admire things about Holland—the way everyone rides bicycles, and no one uses plastic bags. All roads have wide bike lanes. They put chocolate on their bread, and old people are everywhere, and their hair isn't dyed.

My hostess has left a book for me, a little hardcover story collection by a Dutch author named A. L. Snijders (pronounced *Snyders*). I begin to read the book, full of these magnificent, one-page stories. Here's just one of the many that I love, in its entirety, called "Because His Wife."

BECAUSE HIS WIFE

The rooster is as old as a crocodile. You can measure the age of the earth by the coverings on his legs, by the look in his eyes, by the wattles under his beak, by his shrinking comb. From a youngster in a burlap bag he has become a priest, *sacerdos, sacerdos*. When he crows, you can hear that death is a catastrophe. Yet this is only part of the myth. Because his wife . . . His wife is a chicken, just as old as he. Brown at one time, but now completely white (I repeat, and I'm not lying, that this chicken has gone from brown to white in her color-changing chicken-life). Long ago she stopped laying eggs. Nature, say the experts, such is nature, it's natural. But now the white chicken has started laying again. The day before yesterday one egg, and yesterday another.

EACH OF HIS very short stories is like a tight little ball of unspent energy. I read one and I can't read anything else for hours. Each story is giving me permission to write this book the way that I want to write it.

Reading Snijders helps me settle down for real and helps me get excited about my own writing. I sleep and read and sleep and read. Then I start to take notes and soon I am writing, and that is when I know, that is when I *always* know, that everything will be all right, even so far away from home. When I start to write, everything will be OK.

What makes a person a writer has little to do with being published (as I once thought). I write because, when I am thrown off-kilter by getting lost in Amsterdam or by a prolonged illness or by life, say, it's coming back to the page that rights my ship.

I AM AWARE too, even in my distress, that being in a new place with all the attendant discomforts of being there is critical to my larger well-being, critical to being really alive. The discomfort means that I am radically aware of my surroundings in a way that I never am back in the States. I am paying attention to every road sign, looking everywhere for milestones that will help me get "home" to Eindhoven. I am reading new writers, and I'm writing material that is quite different from anything I've written before. The discomfort seems an essential ingredient in this burst of creativity. Being on foreign soil and away from my cozy, happy life seems good for my work, as well as for my humanity, and my understanding of myself.

WHEN THE TIME comes for me to return to America, I am ready, ready to fall back into the blankets in our farmhouse, ready to listen to Craig's voice as he reads me to sleep, ready to wake up where I know all of the street names and the language, and where I never have to pay attention because it is home. But I am not frantic to leave Amsterdam. I am not anxious to leave, as I was at first. In fact, I've made a little life for myself that I could sustain if I wanted to. I am not fleeing Holland for New Jersey, as I would have been if I'd left early. No. It's time to go home, but I feel, even as my plane is taking off, that I will be back.

EIGHTY

The Past Is Never Over

It's forever after the surgery, months after Holland, and I am feeling good, like 92 percent of where I was before I got sick.

Craig and I are invited to a memorial service that's being held at a museum in New Jersey. Our friend who has died is being celebrated by her children and grandchildren. I sit next to Craig on folding chairs in one of the exhibit rooms of the museum. We're holding hands and loving this family, each of whom is taking the lectern and telling us how Pat affected their lives, made them all stronger and kinder. It's magnificent.

There is a reception afterward down in one of the museum's gathering spaces, lit by the sun filtering through the skylights. I am open and emotional and feeling so close to Craig, who shares my feeling about this woman who has died. It is lovely to be with her family, to see how one person can matter in such a profound way, and how, even after her death, we are still getting to know her.

A woman I don't know, who is herself elderly, maybe eighty, comes up to me by the flowers we've helped arrange in vases on all of the tables. She spoke quite eloquently just minutes before, and I tell her how great she was. She asks me, "Have you been blessed with children?" It catches me up short. Until that second, my heart was completely open, but the nosiness of the question and the implications of the phrasing put me immediately on guard. Craig is not with me and I say, feeling trapped, "No, I was not blessed with children." I feel such a wave of unexpected sorrow that I am stunned. This woman, this person whom I've never met before, whose name I don't even know, shakes her head with a look of pity mixed with superiority because she clearly *has* been blessed, and says, "Oh! Well! You should adopt. Why don't you adopt?" She squeezes my bicep and I freeze. I don't like being touched. I look around for Craig. He is chatting with a group of guys and not looking my way. I don't know what to say, nor how a person ought to respond, and the truth is, there are endless reasons and no reasons why we never adopted, and who are you, anyway, I want to say, but don't.

I stand still for a minute. In fact, I am so still, standing there with my mouth open, paused, that I imagine the whole room turning to look, but of course no one does. She fills the silence then. "A dog at least. You should at least adopt a dog." I say something lame like, "Oh excuse me for just a second," and I go and stand on the other side of the room until Craig finds me.

I had really thought that I was over it all, really thought that having fully grieved the miscarriages and the childlessness I was OK. I *have* been OK in fact. But of course grief is not linear, and I should know better than to think it is. Craig and I get home, and just like years and years before when I'd heard a good friend was pregnant, I lie down on the kitchen floor and sob as if I had just heard for the first time, as if it had only just dawned on me that I would never have kids, that my father would die, that my uterus would be cut away, and that the world will move on without me.

As Faulkner wrote, "The past is never dead. It's not even past."

I stand up and, keeping one hand on the wall, I get upstairs, and go to bed that evening at 5:00 p.m., sinking into the seed of grief that just reblossomed, that I didn't know was there.

EIGHTY-ONE

Claude, the Abbey, and the Feral Cat

I go to YouTube to find videos of hatching praying mantis eggs because I want to know what to look for when Claude's eggs finally hatch and his progeny begin their lives in our yard.

I check on Claude's egg sac in the azalea bush every warm day in April, and then every single day in May. I end up missing the hour in which they all swarm out. This happens, the literature says. The egg casing looks fundamentally the same before and after the babies have flown the coop, but they must have hatched by now. Even so I continue to watch the egg sac just in case, until one day there is a daddy long legs (which is not technically a spider, I learn when I look him up), and he has dug a little hole in the abandoned egg sac and his body is in it. Interesting that he is taking over a spent mantid egg sac. Cool. I guess they hatched out when I wasn't there.

I go ahead with the garden, planting my two flats of zinnias (State Fair variety, nice for bouquets) and the rosemary, mint, and parsley. I will keep an eye peeled for baby Claudes this summer. I will look for a praying mantis or two in the sunroom, in the azalea bush where the old egg sac still clings to the bottom-side of an already-bloomed branch. Claude's given me this other reason to be outside—to look for his babies, to watch them keep the aphids from eating my cucumber plants, which I haven't put in yet. But I will. I will.

I haven't walked to the abbey since winter really hit, haven't kept track of anything in my calendar except for appointments. But now that things are warming up I plan to. I want to climb the big hill and see if the little pile of stones is still there by the side of the road.

I will be tremendously glad to clap eyes on the monks, even though they are not chatty, even though I am awkward in situations like that. When I do see them, I will chatter too much out of nervousness, and they will likely not chat enough, for the same reason. But I'll be glad to see the monks, and the baby praying mantids too. I'll be glad to confirm that we have all wandered through into another year, another spring.

The feral cat has not come back. It's spring and the winter was mild, and I hope he's muddled through.

Spring is full of hopping mice and tiny wild rabbits for him to eat if he can catch them. I see moles pushing up the lawn (or rather, I see the pushed-up lawn and assume the moles). I see robins and chickadees hopping inside the lilac hedge. I hope that when the feral cat came to his corner, he found a way to turn it and follow it into this year.

EIGHTY-TWO

Storing Up Beauty

It's summer now, nine or ten months since surgery. I am lying in the hammock looking up at the blue sky behind the leaves of our maple tree and thinking about Grandma Hastings and her cane. I remember her waggling it at me when I was little, saying with a grin, "I'm an ooooold lady." I returned my walking stick to its owner, what, more than six months ago now.

From the hammock I see that the sun is shining hotly on the red geranium by the porch. I notice too the way a hummingbird zigzags through an aimless cloud of midges, finding its way to the bee balm. I lie there, another unread book open on my chest (you'd think I never actually read anything), taking it all in, the hum of the bees in the goosenecked loosestrife, the shimmy of the hammock when I move and settle.

I wish that Warren were still alive. If he were here, he could tell me what kind of frog is making that racket down by Domer Pond. He could point up at the sky and explain how the underwing of a turkey vulture is different from that of a hawk, an eagle, a peregrine falcon.

Later this summer, I will bend to snip mint in my garden and will see, beneath a leaf, the tiniest, bright green praying mantis the size of my pinky nail. Later still, I will be walking to my car, feeling well enough that I'm not even thinking about how well I feel, and out from under the tires will run, not the black and orange feral cat, but a likeness of him. I'll wonder if the light is playing a trick. This cat is white and orange, not black and orange, but the face is unmistakable, the ugly beauty, the stripe down the middle. It is my feral cat's offspring. My feral cat has cast his line into the future, and as I get into the car I sit for a moment before latching my seat belt, breathless with relief. The praying mantis babies, and the new young cat, all set loose in the wild to find their way into the future. And me too. I'm finding a way to cast my own line.

(Later, on a warm October day, I will wash my sheets and hang them on the line, the last load of laundry that will likely be wind dried this year. I will visit Claude's old egg sac on the azalea branch, and there it will be, half missing, but the top of it still glued to its branch by some miracle of adhesion. Because the branches are almost bare, I will be able to see a brand-new egg sac just a few twigs from where Claude's was placed. It's a bit larger, and a bit higher up than Claude's was. Claude's grandbabies will come in the spring.)

MY FATHER HAD his regrets about not learning to play the piano. My regrets thin out but never go completely away. I wasn't able to make Craig a father, and I would have liked to have been a mother too, of course, never mind that I have traded one kind of legacy building for another. I have books now that I shepherd into the world. They are not identical things, having children and writing books, but like a man with a crutch, I hobble along with what I have. Isn't leaving behind a book or two legacy enough? What is the right amount to leave behind to buy ourselves a place in the human race?

My grandmother's name was Rosina West Hastings. She was able to recognize typhoid under a microscope. She told me stories about a curl of smoke to help me sleep, her gray hair unwound down to her waist in the moonlight. She had weeks of "black despair." She loved and lost a man named Horton. Grandma Hastings was my best friend for one year. Since I don't have a child to hold these stories, here . . . I hand them to you.

I stand with a crowd of ghosts at my back.

For now I sway in the hammock, the woman next door calling to her chickens. The monks in the abbey down the road are hauling a bell up a ladder for their bell tower. They are hefting bricks into a dumpster. Next spring, and every spring, will pull the sap up the maple trees, and then the rhubarb leaves will uncrumple. Summer will bring the loosestrife and the clicking dragonflies, the Queen Anne's lace by the side of the road, the blue chicory, along with the banjo-ing bullfrogs. And who can tell what wonders every autumn will bring.

I've come to understand that there is a kind of storing up of beauty, an accumulation of memory, and I know that one day I will lean on my memory of today's loosestrife, laden with fat bees. I will lean on the memory of the hammock rocking me through the dragonfly-filled air of this one July. This moment will give me pleasure later, countless times. Grandma Hastings will be with me forever.

Epilogue

Our pond has a willow tree growing at its edge, and Rosie, the little black cat from when we first moved here, is buried there now. There's one window in the house high enough to look down on the pond. In summer I can't see the water at all, hidden behind the willow's pale leaves, but in winter, I can see through the bare branches of the willow to where Craig skates slowly, using his hockey stick to push a tiny black puck back and forth across the ice. The way I feel about Craig when I look down at him there, so far away from me, brings me to my knees. It's a love made up of the things we couldn't give to one another, but also full of how hard we tried.

I thought Craig would eventually stop holding up the edge of the blanket for me, that it was a courtship thing, but it's been years now and he still does it. He lifts the corner of the blanket for me at night and reveals the heartbeat of our small world, lets the cold air rush under the covers for a moment while I climb into that one spot on earth that is mine.

Acknowledgments

THE VIRGINIA CENTER for the Creative Arts, MacDowell, and Cill Rialaig Arts Centre all supported my work, gave me a place to write, and changed my life.

Mels, Marielle, and Quirijn gave me their home in Holland, where the first draft of this book was written. They also introduced me to the work of A. L. Snijders.

Rosemary James suggested I submit an early draft of this book to the Faulkner-Wisdom Competition. Zachary Lazar was the judge who awarded it the gold medal. Joe de Salvo, who just recently died, was my ideal reader. All three were profoundly encouraging.

Finding the right agent happened because of friends like Sugi Ganeshananthan, Tina Shmerler, and Ellen Marie Wiseman. My agent, Michael Carr at Veritas, has turned out to be a kindred spirit. This book would not have found its perfect home at Algonquin without him.

Amy Gash, my editor at Algonquin, is brilliant, generous, and hilarious. To have this book land at Algonquin, and with Amy, seems too good to be true, but it's true nonetheless.

Peter Wattley built my writing space. His artistry, gentle spirit, and friendship infuse the place.

David Ebenbach is a good friend and a trusted reader. He was the first to read this book in its earliest incarnation, and cheered me on, as he does. Sian Gibby also helped with an early draft, along with members of the Three Birds Writing Group, Joseph Eveld and Courtni Jeffers. Marie Myung-Ok Lee is a brilliant, generous writer and friend whose presence in my life makes me a better human being and writer.

I have known Shay Craig, Daniel DaSilva, and Jennifer Grant Scopes for most of my life. They are there when my 3:00 a.m. mind awakens to silly devastations. What would I do without them?

For the first twelve years of my life, my parents read to me every night. They gave me a filing cabinet when I was seven, and a typewriter when I was nine. In third grade, after begging, they allowed me to wear my glasses on a chain around my neck, just like my teacher, Mrs. Gloger. Mom and Dad supported the writer in me before I even understood what that meant.

Zonker the one-eyed cat in this book continues on. Every night as he settles down near me in bed, I ask him to please live forever.

And finally, everything good and happy in my life begins and ends with Craig.